D0852019

drybar®

GOOD HAIR FOR ALL

THE drybar GUIDE TO
GOOD HAIR FOR ALL

Alli Webb
WITH CRYSTAL MEERS

ABRAMS, NEW YORK

EDITOR: Rebecca Kaplan
DESIGNER: Jenny Kraemer
ART DIRECTOR: Andrea Rell
PRODUCTION MANAGER: Denise LaCongo

Library of Congress Control Number: 2015956325

ISBN: 978-1-4197-2106-9

Printed and bound in the United States
10 9 8 7 6 5 4 3 2 1

Abrams Image books are available at special discounts when purchased in quantity for premiums and promotions as well as fundraising or educational use. Special editions can also be created to specification. For details, contact specialsales@abramsbooks.com or the address below.

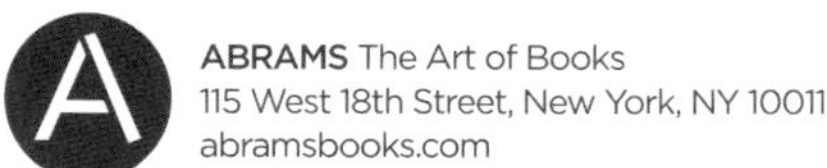

My mom...

absolutely adored reading and spent a lifetime trying to get me to fall in love with books. However, hair was always my passion, and while my mom didn't love it the way I did, she happily blew out my curly hair all the time. As a young girl, I was so lucky to have such a supportive mother who always encouraged me to follow my dreams.

I'll never forget how excited she was when she learned her very own daughter was writing a book. While I can't share this book with her, I can dedicate it to her. So here goes:

Mom, wherever you are, I thank you and I love you. I would not be the woman I am today without your unwavering love and patience. This book is my gift to you.

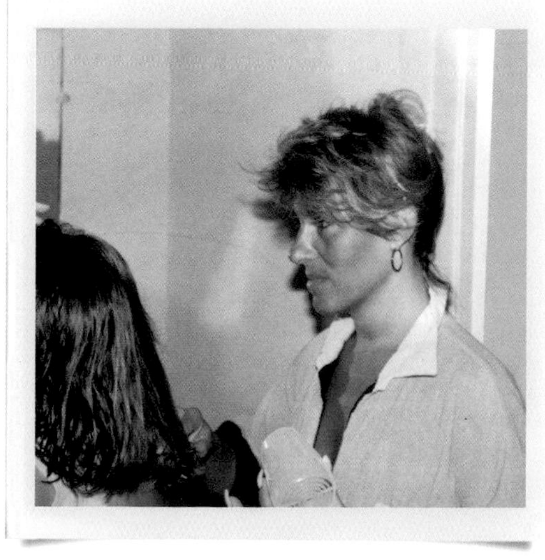

Rozi Landau 10/16/1950–1/29/2016.
Alli & Rozi 1984 Hollywood, FL

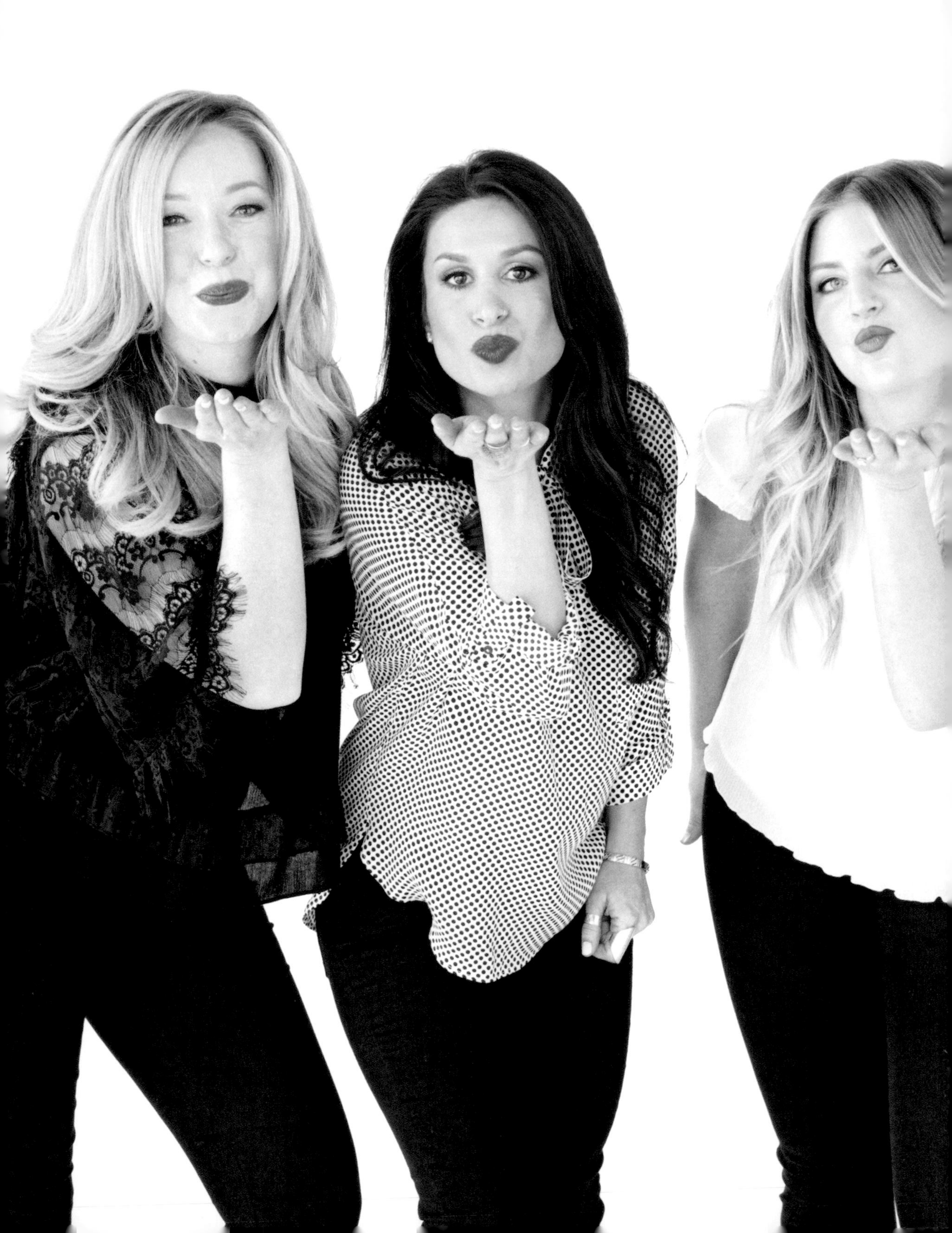

CONTENTS

9 INTRODUCTION

A Girl and Her Blow-Dryer: The Alli Webb Story

14 **What is Drybar?**

18 **Aperitif:** Make Every Day a Good (Hair) Day

21 SECTION 1

Prep School: Everything You Need to Know about Your Hair (IMHO)

31 SECTION 2

Bag of Tricks: The Tools You'll Need for Making Your Own Drybar Magic

43 SECTION 3

Hey, Good Lookin': Drybar's Signature Styles

49 **The Straight Up**
Straight with a Little Bit of Body

59 **The Manhattan**
Sleek and Smooth

69 **The Cosmo**
Lots of Loose Curls

79 **The Mai Tai**
Messy, Beachy Hair

89 **The Cosmo-Tai**
A Little Cosmo, a Little Mai Tai

99 **The Dirty Martini**
Tousled and Textured

109 **The Southern Comfort**
Big Hair, Lots of Volume

120 SECTION 4

Beyond the Blowout: Other Styles to Know and Love

123 **The Perfect Pony**
To the Gym and Back

129 **The Fun Bun**
Not Just for Bad Hair Days

135 **The Barmaid Braid**
AKA What Bangs?

141 SECTION 5

After Party: Making Your Look Last

147 **The Dry Tai**
AKA The Mai Tai in a Minute

153 **The Straighter Up**
Second-Day Hair, Served Neat

159 SECTION 6

Q & A Session (Questions & Alli)

166 10 Core Values

168 **Thank You**

174 **Acknowledgments**

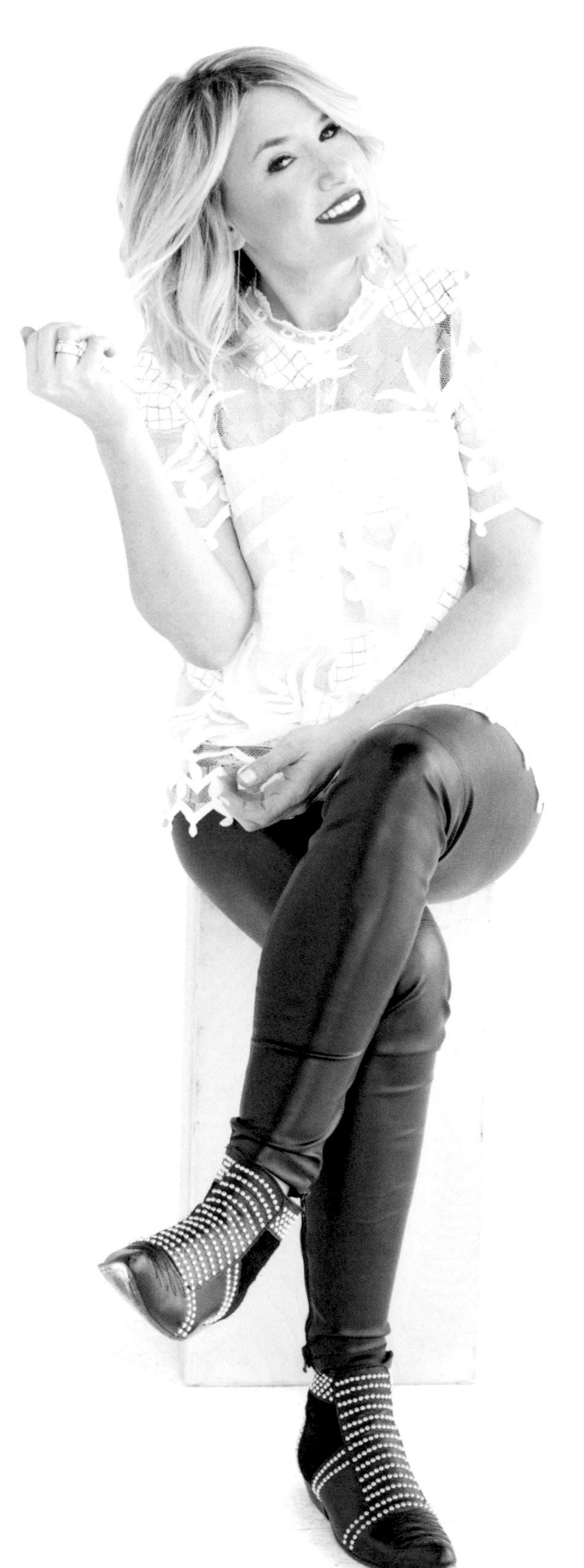

INTRODUCTION

A GIRL AND HER BLOW-DRYER: THE ALLI WEBB STORY

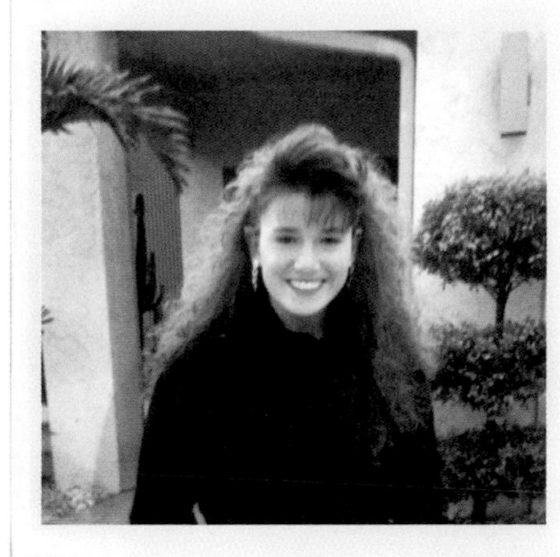

Alli, 1988
Boca Raton, FL

Yep, that's me. Back then, I was Alli, the girl with the crazy, impossible, unruly, super-duper, totally uncool curly hair.

At least, that's how I felt.

I know, I know. It might not look that bananas to you. It just looks like hair. But trust me, waking up with a wild nest on top of your head in a world where supermodels like Christie Brinkley and Cindy Crawford were the hair idols of the day was enough to make anyone want to stay in bed. Some nights, I would struggle for hours before bed. If I blew out my hair, then slept on it, it would surely have to be less frizzy when I woke up, right? Wrong. Most mornings before school, I would lock myself in the bathroom with brush and blow-dryer until my brother banged on the door, yelling for me to get out. Some days, my hair semi-cooperated before I left the house. Other days, I threw it in a bun. Most days—even when I had a really cute outfit on!—I felt as if my pursuit of having even one good hair day was a complete and utter lost cause.

How did those shampoo-commercial girls get that freaking hair? It was a conundrum to me. Seriously. Bouncy hair became one of life's great mysteries—something only the secret society of professional hairdressers knew about. I tried every product I could get my hands on and experimented with every brush under the sun. I washed my hair in the morning and pulled it into taut braids to get it to de-frizz. I deep-conditioned it at night and slept on it in hopes this would help calm it down. I listened to old wives' tales, clipped tips out of magazines, and even ironed my hair with an actual iron, the kind used for clothes.

As I got older, I started going to the beauty parlor with my mom (who passed down her obsession with beauty and being perfectly put together at all times) when she got her hair, nails, and toes done. A giant lightbulb, or, in my case, a bright yellow blow-dryer, went on: If I was going to figure out how to do my own hair, I was going to need to get a job at a salon. I started as a receptionist at the salon at the mall a few weeks later—shout-out to Town Center for all my fellow Boca Raton ladies. My hair never looked better. One of the perks (the ultimate perk!) was that the stylists there would blow out my hair all the time. Hello! Best. Job. Ever. Every shift, I answered the phones, booked appointments, swept the floors, and asked (OK, stalked) the stylists for their secrets on what to do with my mop. I studied, I practiced, and I tried every technique they showed me. After living with wild and unruly hair all my life, I finally started to feel as though I was on the brink of cracking the pretty-hair code.

"AFTER LIVING WITH WILD AND UNRULY HAIR ALL MY LIFE, I FINALLY STARTED TO FEEL AS THOUGH I WAS ON THE BRINK OF CRACKING THE PRETTY-HAIR CODE."

From that moment on, I knew I wanted to pursue my dream of becoming a hairstylist. It took me a few years, but after a slew of other jobs (and a lot of encouragement from my brother, and now business partner, Michael Landau), I eventually followed my heart and enrolled in beauty school in Boca. There I had the great honor of assisting John Peters, who taught me not only so much about hair but also how to really connect with clients and how to run a successful salon. With a solid foundation and my cosmetology certification in hand, I headed for New York City. I landed a job at John Sahag's salon—the only salon where I wanted to work because the man himself was beyond famous for his dry styling. There I began assisting some of the most respected hairstylists in the industry. I soaked up every tip and technique I could and even started coming up with some of my own. It seemed as if everyone had a new tool, a new style, and a new way to get the job done (after twenty years of styling hair, I'm still picking up new tricks from the stylists at Drybar). I wanted to break the art of a good blowout down to a science so I could get—and give—the perfect blowout every time.

Somewhere along the way, I met Cameron Webb. (OK, of course I remember the exact moment, in the exact place, at the exact time—we totally locked eyes from across the room at a bar named Hell in the Meatpacking District thirteen years ago. I'll tell you the story sometime.) We fell in love, got married, and moved to Southern California, where we had our two boys, Grant Charles and Kit Hucklebee. For the next five years, I was seriously in the mom zone. And while I didn't stop doing hair altogether, I did it on my own terms in a way that worked for me and my family.

One sunny Southern California day, I decided to post a note on a popular mommy blog for my mobile blow-dry business, Straight-at-Home. Soon I was driving all over LA to all the mommies I knew, blowing out their hair while their babies napped. It was perfect, but I quickly found myself with a good problem: I had way more clients than I had time. It turned out that women had only two not-so-great

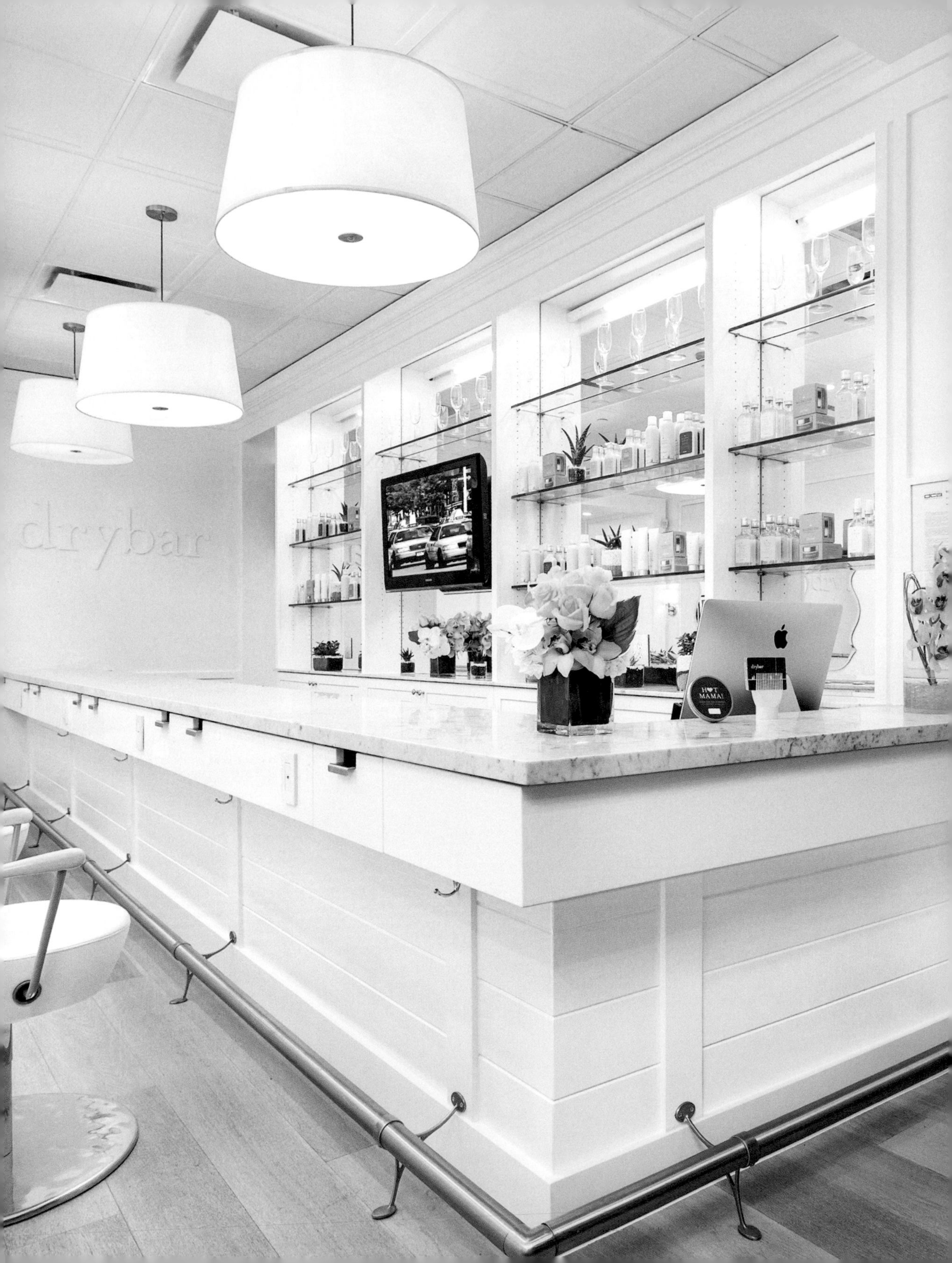
drybar

The first Drybar shop opened in February 2010 in Brentwood, CA.

choices out there when it came to getting a blowout: a traditional full-service salon, where blowouts are super expensive and most stylists really prefer doing cut and color, or the discount chain, where women suffer through a speedy, no-frills experience. There really wasn't a good option for women like me, who longed for a great blowout in a fun and beautiful setting. It didn't take me long to see that women would get a lot more blowouts if it was fun and easy, and if the price was right. I also realized that if I didn't have to waste so many hours schlepping around in the car, I would have more time for clients. That's when I knew I needed to bring my mobile business to life in a brick-and-mortar way.

Naturally, I went to my husband, Cameron, and my brother, Michael, first. Cam loved the idea right off the bat! He would always say, "You get your nails done once a week, and I never really notice, but whenever you get a blowout, it's the first thing I see!" Michael took a bit more convincing, not only because he's bald, but also because he's married to Sarah, a gorgeous woman whose perfect, naturally straight locks never really need a blowout (though she would eventually become Drybar's director of team member experience and in-house DJ). But, you guessed it, everyone got on board, and that is how Drybar was born.

WHAT IS DRYBAR?

If you're never been to a Drybar, you're probably scratching your head right now. Some people say it's a blowdry bar. Others say it's a revolution. Call it what you want, but to me it's a happy place, a refuge, a healthy addiction, and a company that brings a smile and confidence to the faces of millions of women of all ages and backgrounds. (A fact that I am enormously humbled by.)

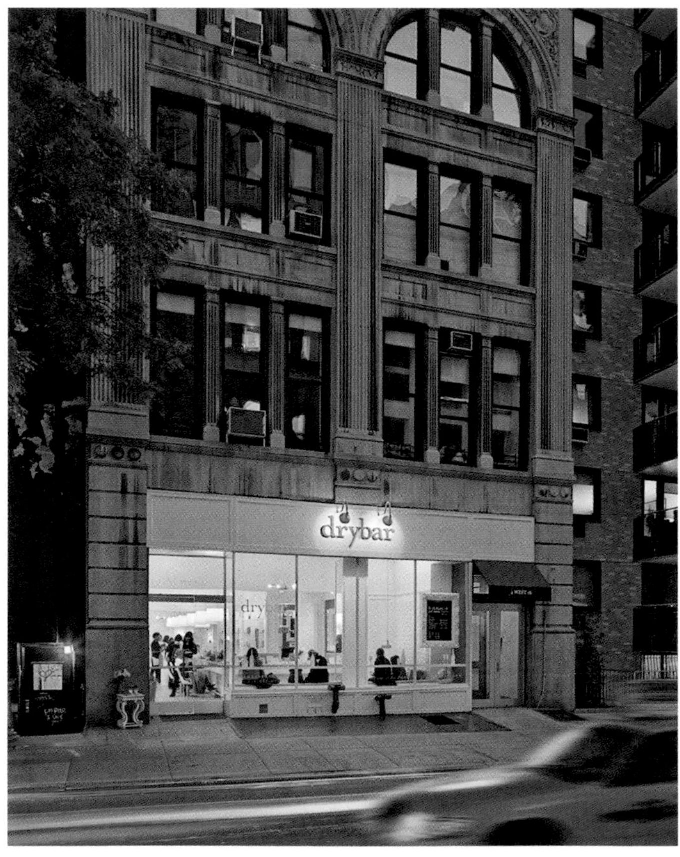

NYC Flagship, Flatiron, opened September 2011.

This shot was taken at our very first (and then only) Drybar location in Brentwood, 2010.

Of our 10 Core Values, one of my very favorites is #10, We Are Family. Drybar was started by this family and anyone who works with us is a part of our family. While we have all played a lot of different roles and worn many hats over the years, there's no one else I'd rather be on this journey with than these three.

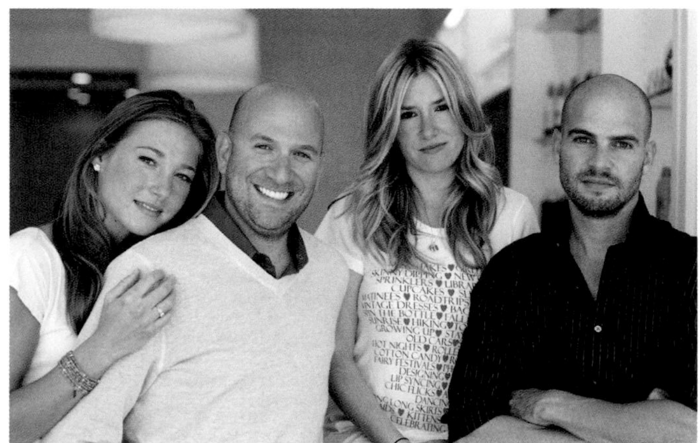

In the fall of 2009, I founded the company with my extraordinarily talented creative-director husband, Cameron, my entrepreneur brother Michael, and his now-wife, Sarah Hutnick.

The very first Drybar location opened in Brentwood, California, in 2010. It was designed by our pal, award-winning architect Josh Heitler. We planned on thirty to forty clients a day. NBD. But the media went wild and the women of Los Angeles even more so. Business quickly exceeded our expectations, nearly doubling our projections from the get-go. In fact, there was so much demand that we had to turn down customers who were attempting to walk in or call in without having booked an appointment via the website. Turning away people made us so sad. (Seriously. So. Sad.) The only answer was to open another location. And another. And another. (If we're not in your town yet, hopefully we will be soon.)

Why? Most men don't really get it. But women do. The ability for a woman to get a pro-quality blowout in a beautiful, upbeat, and comfortable setting at an affordable price was groundbreaking. Our success comes from how easily and deeply Drybar becomes interwoven into the lives of so many women.

By 2011 we had solidly proven the idea in LA. But what about everywhere else? Would it work coast-to-coast, so that ladies on the go could get the same great Drybar blowout in New York as in Los Angeles, as in Chicago, as in Dallas, etc.? In a word, YES. The company's launch in New York was a raging success. And with that boost of confidence, Drybar quickly planted flags in Chicago, Dallas, Boston, Washington, DC, San Francisco, Phoenix, San Diego, Houston, Atlanta, and other cities. Ladies in all of these markets embraced us with giddiness.

Today, Drybar operates 60 locations, employs more than 3,000 people, produces a wildly popular line of styling products and tools sold in their shops and at Sephora, Nordstrom, Bloomingdales, and Ulta Beauty. We're growing ever day thanks to the help of many talented executives, managers, and creative-types.

Still, at the heart of it all is really great hair. Our family of stylists is constantly trained on the finer points of the perfect blowout. The weekend clients hit the town or a wedding with a bounce in their step. The weekday regulars settle in to be pampered as part of their routine. Businesswomen claim that the confidence spike that follows a great blowout can change their entire workweek. In fact, some of the most loyal clients have vowed to never again wash their own hair. And believe it or not, we are just getting started. Drybar has yet to launch in Europe or Asia (there are a bunch of women there, by the way). We'll go anywhere in pursuit of good hair.

Even after opening all of our shops, launching a full line of products and tools, training thousands of stylists, answering countless questions, and giving millions (literally millions) of blowouts, I'm still learning how to handle my curls—and have spent some serious quality time with every other type of hair under the sun. And since we don't have a Drybar everywhere (yet), think of this book as the definitive how-to guide to achieving the very best blowouts and hair styles you can at home. I'm so excited to share everything I've picked up during my lifelong pursuit of good hair.

First, let's identify your hair type and the issues you may have going on and brush up (pun intended—be prepared for a few of those!) on the essential products and tools that you'll want to have within reach. Then I'll take you step-by-step through the blowout basics of our styles at Drybar, the same way we do with the thousands of stylists in our Drybar fam. There are tons of dos and don'ts to go over, loads of tips on how to care for your hair and even on what to do when there's not a blow-dryer or curling iron in sight.

Drybar stands for good hair for all. Allow me to show you how it's done.

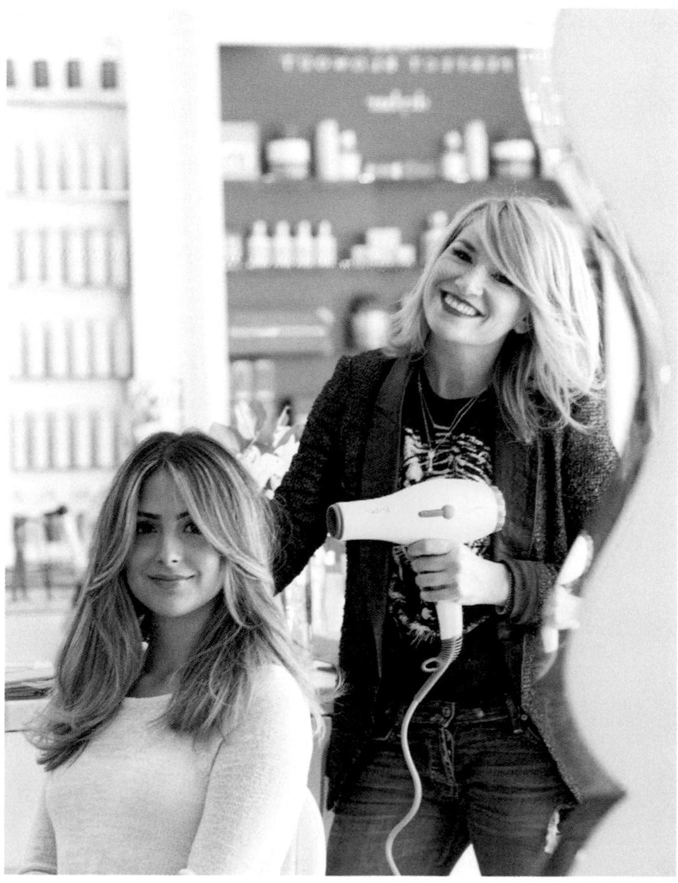

APERITIF

MAKE EVERY DAY A GOOD (HAIR) DAY

One of the earliest life lessons I learned was that when I look good, I feel good. And for me, that is (almost) all about my hair.

Now, mind you, this was when I was, like, ten.

And, yep, it's still true today.

Tell me if this sounds familiar: You wake up and evaluate your hair while brushing your teeth. If it's good, there might be an equally good outfit in your future, followed by maybe your favorite lipstick, possibly a fancy coffee, and perhaps a few highly caffeinated texts to your favorite people telling them how much you love them and to have a great day. If it's bad, there are two options: Either you get a handle on the situation by taking a shower (i.e., starting over) or the question becomes ponytail or bun, and the chances of throwing on a sweatshirt skyrocket, you order a black coffee to go with your sunglasses on, and the only thing anyone is getting out of you is an emoticon—or maaaaaybe a popular meme with a grouchy 'tude. Maybe.

See? Bad hair days are just bummers. They have an impact on everything you do. Personally, I know that when I'm not thinking about/messing with/worrying about/hating on my hair, I have more time and energy to be a better mom, a nicer wife, a more considerate business partner (or less bratty little sister, depending on who you ask), a more present friend, and just an easier person to deal with in general. There's no denying that the way I feel—whether that's happy, sad, frustrated, mad, or otherwise—has a huge part to play in how I act. A blowout just happens to be the magic ticket for me (and, well, for millions of Drybar clients across the country and zillions of curly-haired people around the world). A recent college study claims 55 percent of women—that's right, more than half!—say they are nicer when their hair looks good.

Back when I was ten, I didn't know how, exactly, to put it into words. I just knew that when I liked my hair, I liked myself, and I liked everything else a whole lot more too. Since then, so many women—especially my mother—have taught me to take good care of myself so that I can feel my best and be my best for others too.

I would never have imagined all those years ago that we could build a business on this notion, but knowing what a difference the right brush and a good blow-dryer made in my life, I was sure there was a good chance that other women felt the same way. I'm proud to say that thousands of ladies practically float out of Drybar on a daily basis with hair that makes them feel amazing, and with confidence to go with it. For years, women have been telling me, tweeting at me, and posting on Facebook and Instagram that Drybar has changed their lives, that they've never felt better than after an appointment at one of our shops, and that they wonder what they ever did before Drybar.

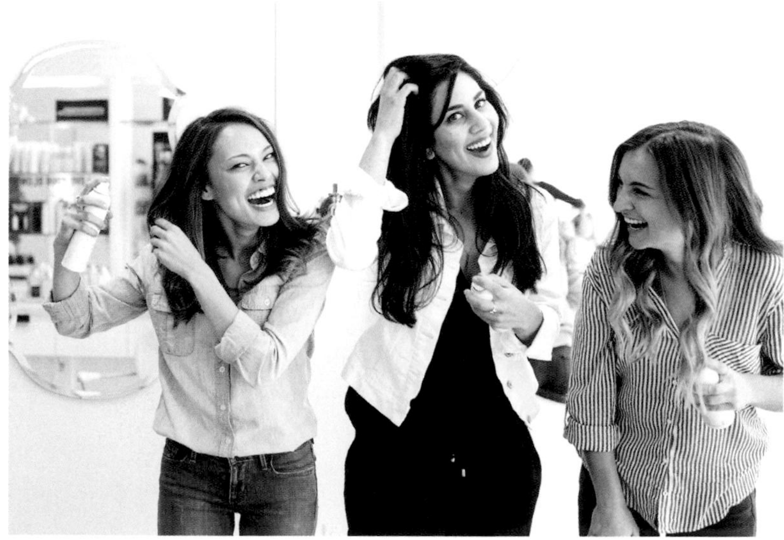

SECTION 1:

PREP SCHOOL

Everything You Need to Know about Your Hair (IMHO)

Hair. We all have it. Well, most of us do (sorry, Michael). Here's the thing: It's all super different. The blonde over there with perfectly straight hair? Maybe her alarm went off while you were still in dreamland, so she had an extra hour before work to get it just right. (Or maybe she went to Drybar at 7 a.m.?!) The brunette with the big bouncy curls? There's a chance she slept in rollers last night—if she slept at all. The woman with the pink textured bob and the perfect bed head? Well, she just woke up like that (but she does do a deep conditioning treatment twice a week and has to touch up her color at least once a month). My point is, even though we all have hair, everyone's is different (thank goodness!). We don't have any control over the mop we were given, but we do have the power to style it however we want and to take care of it as best we can. Be good to your hair, and it will be good to you.

BEAUTY SCHOOL: WHAT IS HAIR, ANYWAY?

Class is now in session (but we will make this quick)!

A little basic anatomy of what's happening on your bod right now: Hair is growing from your follicles. What's a follicle? You have millions of these tiny little things all over that basically produce hair. The part of each strand that is above the skin's surface is the shaft, below the surface is the root, and at the base of that root is the blub. Attached to the bulb, you've got a dermal papilla (that's where the hair bulb picks up nutrients and good stuff to generate new cells), a sebaceous gland (basically an oil factory), and the arrector pili (a teeny muscle that contracts when you are freezing or freaked out ala goosebumps). New cells come from the papilla. As they die (RIP), they move up and out of the follicle, and as they do they smush together to form keratin, the protein that makes up most of the hair shaft (oh, and your fingernails are mostly keratin too!). Pretty interesting, right?

Each strand of hair is a universe of its own. The protective outside layer is called the cuticle and it's made up of layers of overlapping scales. Getting the cuticle to lie flat is the secret to smooth, silky hair. Underneath the cuticle is the cortex, which is mostly long chains of amino acids (think protein fibers twisted up like a rope) that gives the hair strand its color and shape. It's also where the side bonds live. Side bonds can be broken by moisture and heat, so when you sleep in braids, use a at iron, or get a perm, that's where the bonds break and reshape and all the action goes down, but it's a good thing—helps us change things up. The stronger and healthier these bonds, the stronger and healthier your hair is. Oh, and in the very center is the medulla. But don't worry about it. It's kinda just there. (No, really. Ask a scientist!)

IDENTIFYING YOUR HAIR TYPE

Even more important than the science behind your hair is really understanding your particular hair type. Why? Because it totally dictates how you should care for and work with your hair. Everyone wants shiny, healthy-looking locks, but how each person gets there is going to be a road of their own. The same moisturizing shampoo that "transformed" your friend's curls may very well leave your hair looking like an oil slick. The texturizing spray that gave your straight hair beachy waves could turn your friend's overprocessed hair into straw. From knowing when to wash and condition to knowing which sort of brush will make your hair dreams come true, it all comes down to hair type.

And it's just as simple as straight, wavy, or curly. Hair texture rules which looks are really going to work for you and which products and tools you'll need to get there (how long it will take really depends on your hair density, or the number of hairs on your head). Your texture is fine, medium, or coarse. A strand of fine hair feels very thin. Coarse hair is thicker, with a rougher cuticle. Medium falls somewhere in the middle and often varies depending on where it is on the scalp (as when someone's hair is stick straight on top and hiding a mess of waves underneath).

BE COOL
Cold rinses are not a myth. A blast of chilly water closes the cuticles of your hair, which is, remember, the key to achieving shiny, happy hair!

HANDLE WITH CARE
When your hair is wet, it's super fragile. The best way to avoid breakage is to detangle it using a wide-tooth comb. Start at the ends and work your way up.

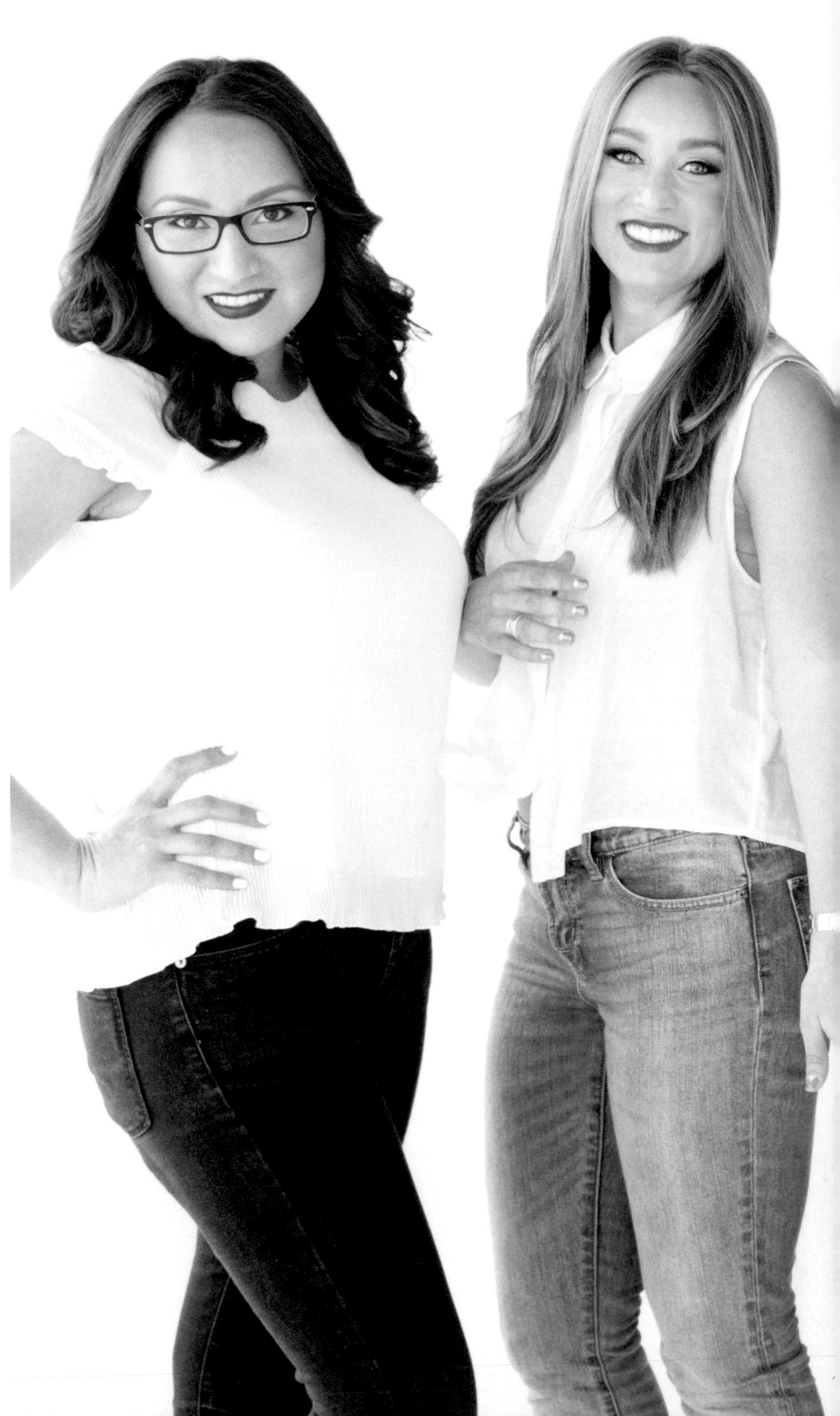

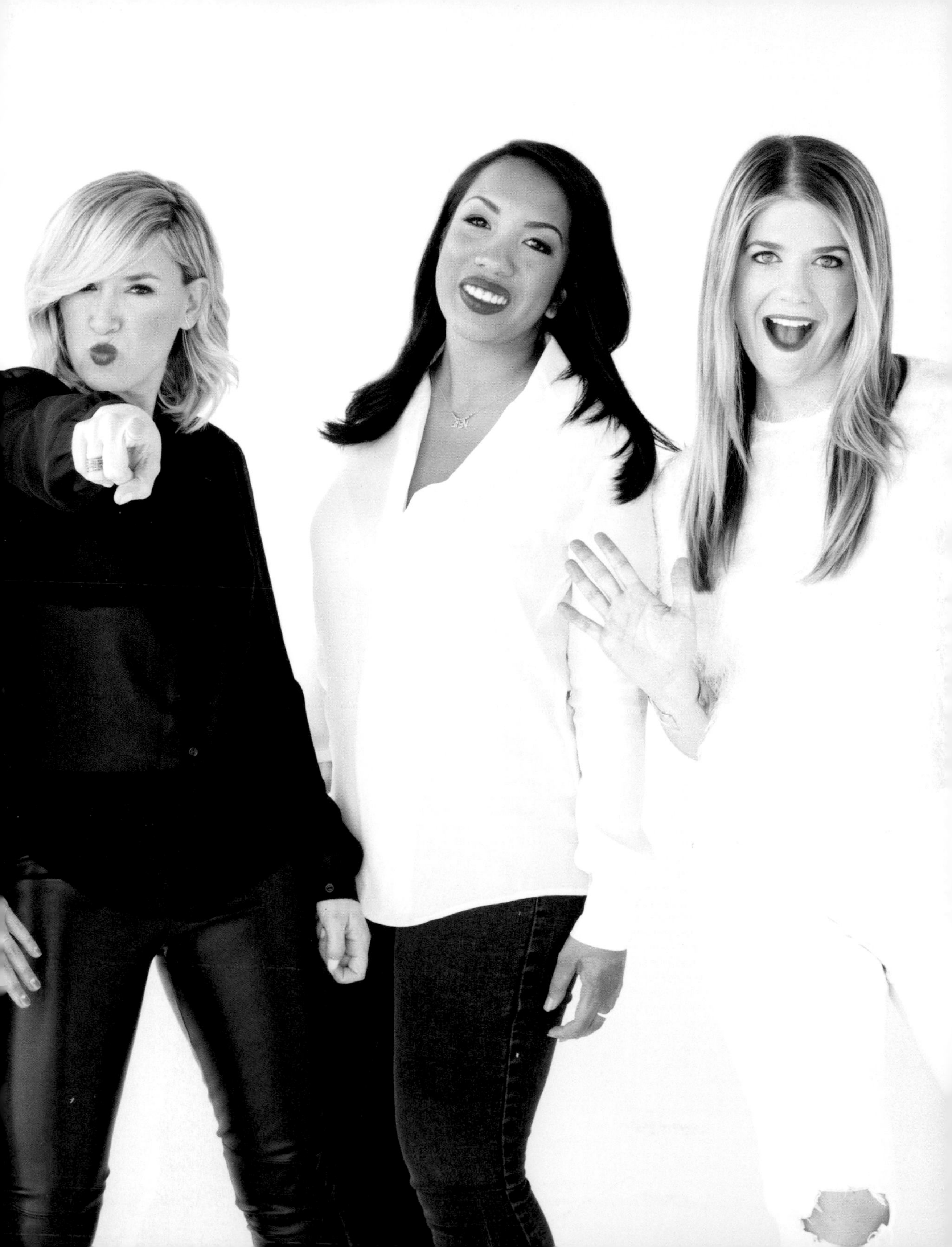

WHAT'S YOUR TYPE?

TO FIGURE OUT YOUR HAIR TYPE
ONCE AND FOR ALL, WASH YOUR HAIR AND LET IT AIR-DRY. TAKE A GOOD LOOK AT YOUR HAIR. ONCE YOU KNOW WHAT YOU'RE WORKING WITH, CHOOSING THE RIGHT PRODUCTS WILL BE A BREEZE.

So what are the options here? After millions (yes, millions) of blowouts at Drybar, we have found the most common hair types are:

Straight and Fine

This is the baby-fine hair that comes to mind when you picture natural blondes from Scandinavia. People with this hair type often feel that their bangs get greasy by the end of the day, and they have a very tough time getting much wave or volume to hold.

Straight and Medium

Yep, this is just what it sounds like: straight hair that's relatively easy to work with and is typically tame, even when it air-dries. This inspires a lot of hair envy in women with trickier hair, but the ladies who have it often complain that their style feels blah.

Straight and Coarse

Most often, this is thick, dense hair—and lots of it. Many of our Asian clients have gorgeous hair that's long and super strong but way resistant to keeping a curl. (PS: I would kill for this hair type!)

Wavy and Medium

This hair type is a mixed bag: Some strands have tons of bend, others seem to have very little. It's not unusual for someone to have totally straight hair on top and a wavy part underneath. It plays well with hot tools.

Wavy and Coarse

Maybe she was born with it, maybe it's the result of a lot of styling or color processing. The cuticle is often pretty rough when it comes to this hair type, so it tends to need a little more TLC and some good products to calm down. It's also very prone to frizz.

Curly and Medium

Think Taylor Swift: She can do a full head of curls one day and smooth, glamorous hair the next. This hair has a lot of natural body and bounce.

Curly and Coarse

Here's where things can get tricky: The cuticles are going every which way and can often become interlocked, so be gentle! These strands are delicate and can easily be damaged by too much heat or by overprocessing—two good things to keep in mind, especially if you have Indian or Persian hair types.

Highly Textured

What makes extremely curly hair so challenging is the fine texture, extreme curl, and potential density—and that's also what makes it prone to breakage. African-American hair often falls into this category. Using high heat and ultra firm tension are a must, along with smaller sections and the right brush size/type. Hydrating cream and oil based products will also help to calm natural texture and make the blowout much easier and faster.

A CLEAN START

There are lots of dos in this book, and a few very important don'ts. The biggest don't is (drumroll, please) don't wash your hair every day. This goes for all hair types and textures, for virgin hair and color-processed locks. It's just not going to do your hair any good. If you're thinking, I have to wash my hair every day, it gets so oily, at least try dry shampoo or even some baby powder—just trust me!

Depending on your hair type, overwashing can actually be part of the problem. It can strip away the natural oils that help strengthen the hair and prevent breakage, or, on the flip side, it can lead to increased oil production—and that's what puts your hair on the fast track to greasy strands.

Washing every other day, or even every three days, is just enough to give your hair the gentle cleansing and moisture boost it needs (a few girls at the Drybar Support Center swear they go a week between washings, and I know there are plenty of our clients who make their blowouts stretch too). If your hair is super fine, try a volumizing shampoo. If it tends to go limp quickly, skip the

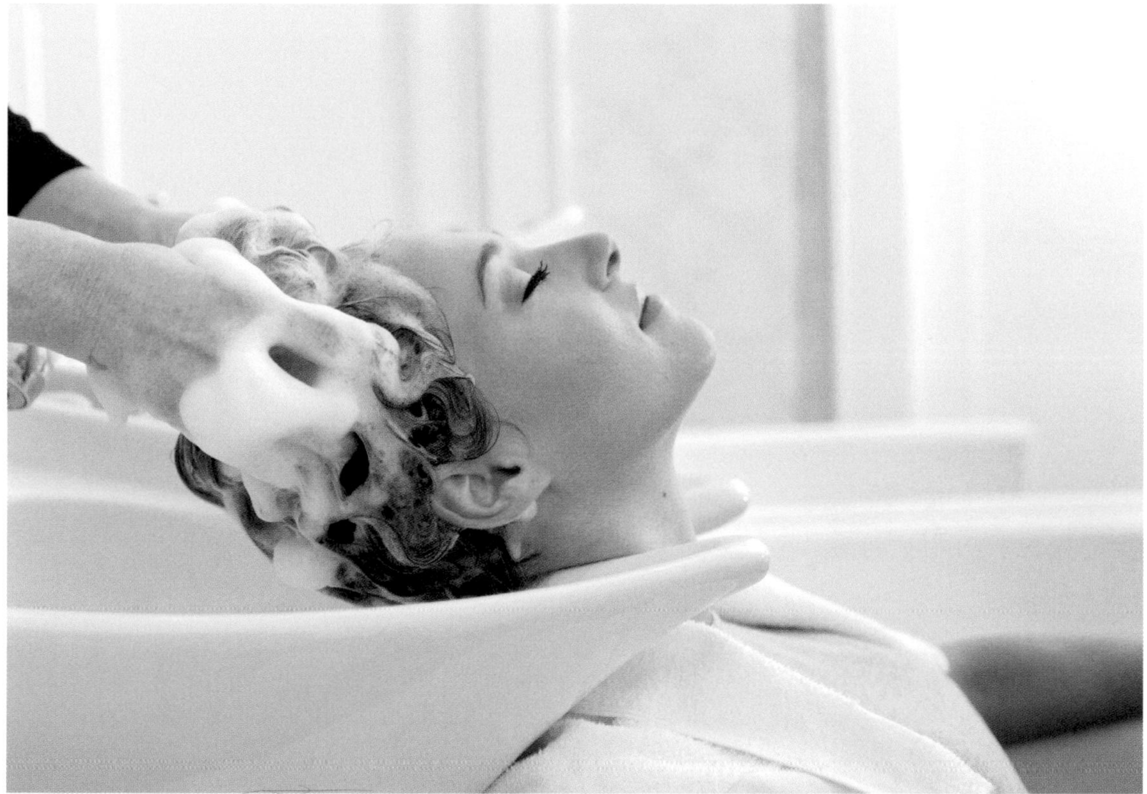

conditioner (it will just weigh you down) or condition just the ends. If your hair is tangly, make sure to use a hydrating conditioner whenever you wash. But if your scalp gets greasy, apply conditioner only from midshaft to ends.

If you insist on washing every single day, promise you'll choose a mild, moisturizing shampoo and a lightweight conditioner? Pinky swear? This way, you'll get the fresh and clean feeling you like without stripping the hair or weighing it down.

SECTION 2:

BAG OF TRICKS

The Tools You'll Need for Making Your Own Drybar Magic

Hair this good doesn't just happen on its own. You'll need the right products and the right tools to get the job done. It might seem like a lot of gear at first, but being prepared will save you loads of frustration (read: fewer wrinkles!). Having the right stuff will not only save you tons of time; it will save the integrity of your hair too. Using the wrong tools or tools that have been poorly made can wind up costing you big-time. If you plan on styling your hair often, it's definitely worth the investment.

Now, there are two essentials that money can't buy:

Time

Give yourself plenty of time. How long? That depends on your hair type, density, and style, and on how much practice you've had doing your hair on your own. But whatever look you're going for, rushing through a blowout is a surefire way to, well, blow it. It takes us pros at Drybar thirty to forty-five minutes to tame the average mane, and we do it all day long. It's safe to assume that it should take you about that long too. The good news is, if you put in the time upfront, your blowout will actually last a few days. On the flip side, rush through it, and your blowout might not last even till lunch.

Practice

When you're styling your hair in a new way for the very first time, it might take a few tries to get it just right. That's totally normal. As you become more familiar with sectioning, handling the brush, and using extras like clips or rollers, the whole process will get easier and you'll move more quickly. You'll be a pro before you know it.

Everything else on our list of must-haves you can find at your local Drybar or beauty shop, or online.

TOOLS

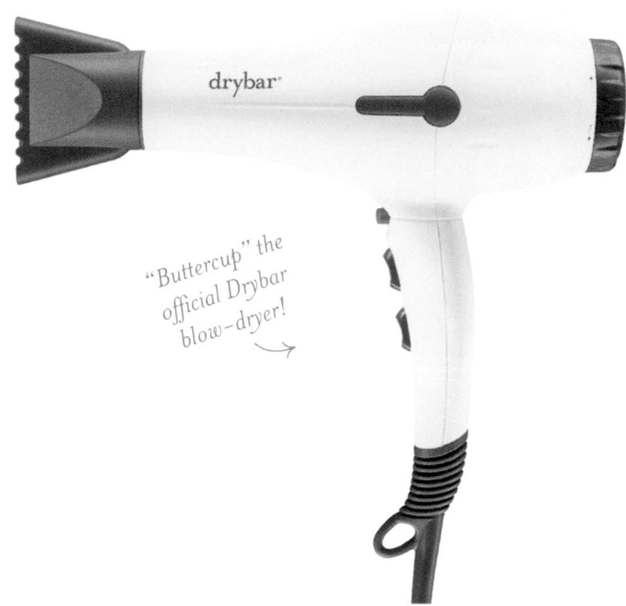

"Buttercup" the official Drybar blow-dryer!

A Good Blow-Dryer

Trying to get a good blowout with a bad blow-dryer is like riding a tricycle across town: You'll eventually get there, but there's definitely a better way to go. A good dryer doesn't mean the most expensive dryer you can find. Look for a machine within your budget that has multiple heat settings, so you can control the temperature, and a cold-shot button for sealing your ends and finishing off your look. Also make sure the dryer is lightweight and comfortable in your hand, and that you can maneuver it well. We all know how tiring it gets holding a blow-dryer above your head! And lastly, look for ionic technology; the negative ions help dry hair faster, to protect your hair from overexposure to heat.

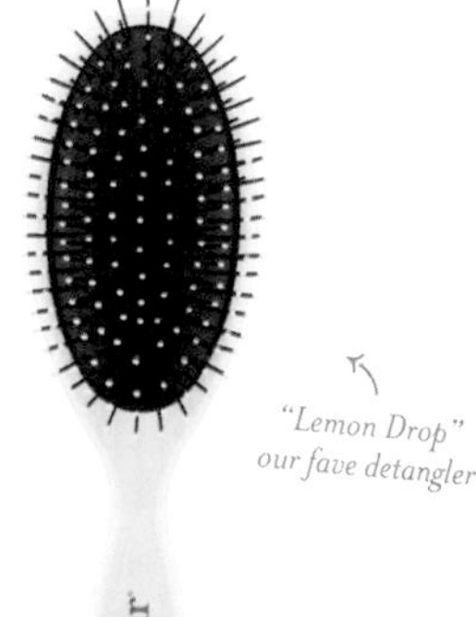

"Lemon Drop" our fave detangler

Detangling Brush

We love our Lemon Drop. Use the detangling brush in the shower or on wet hair. Its cushioned bristles have lots of give, so they can get the knots out without breaking the hair.

Wide-Tooth Comb

This is a great tool for detangling your hair while it's wet or dry. It also comes in handy for parting and sectioning.

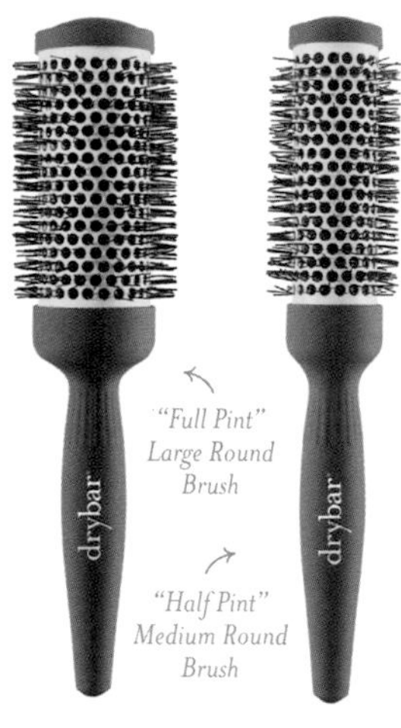

"Full Pint" Large Round Brush

"Half Pint" Medium Round Brush

Round Ceramic-Barrel Brush

Round brushes are essential to styling. They help give the hair direction and movement. For best results, look for brushes with ceramic barrels. The air from your blow-dryer heats up the barrel of the brush, which helps to smooth the cuticle even faster. These brushes really help lock in curl and volume, and add shine. They're a total must-have, in my book.

You may want to keep a few different-size brushes around:

- A small round ceramic-barrel brush for shorter hair or tighter curls.
- A medium round ceramic barrel brush for giving loose curls and/or waves, straightening short to medium-length hair, and great for bangs.
- A large barrel brush for adding body and wave in long hair or for straightening shoulder-length hair.

Round Boar-Bristle Brush

These are classic and come in a variety of sizes. Awesome for when you need to really get in at your scalp to smooth roots or curly/coarse hair. The bristles help evenly distribute the natural oils from your scalp, to help make hair shiny and smooth.

Our "Hold Me" hair clips

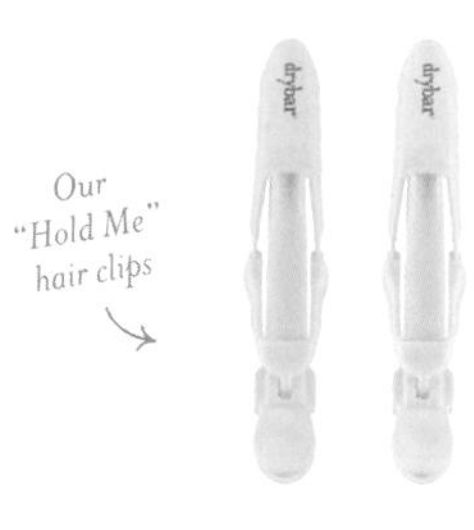

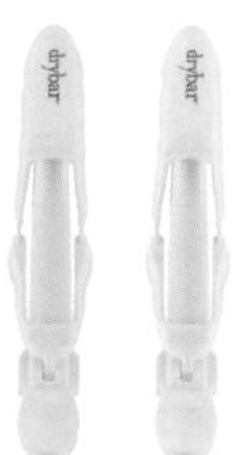

Clips

Meet the unsung hero of your styling kit! Clips like the Hold Me Hair Clips can be used to cleanly section hair and to hold hair—wet or dry—in place. Just four of these clips will make your life so much better. I swear!

Mirror

Any mirror where you can get a look at your pretty self will do, but styling will be extra easy if you can set up a second mirror that will allow you to see the back of your head. Personally, I searched all over the place until I found one I could install in my bathroom that rotates off the wall so I can see the back and the crown of my head. You do not have to do this. I'm nuts (and may be under more pressure than most to have good hair all the time). A handheld mirror totally works. PS: Your cell phone does the trick too in a pinch.

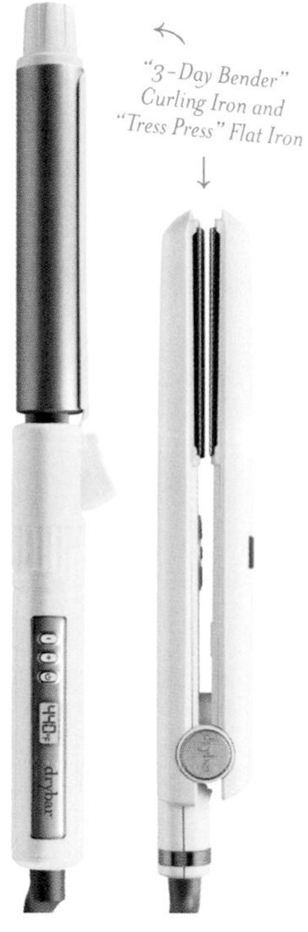

"3-Day Bender" Curling Iron and "Tress Press" Flat Iron

Curling Iron

This is a must-have for defining your natural curls or creating new ones. Our 3-Day-Bender curling iron has a rotating clamp that makes it super easy to manipulate the hair. Ideally, a curling iron should heat up fast and have multiple settings up to 450°F (230°C). Always preheat your curling iron: The higher the heat, the less time you'll need to set your hair. If you have very fragile hair, go with a lower heat setting, around 350°F (175°C).

Flat Iron

A flat iron is key for creating sleek, straight styles or smoothing frizzy pieces. You can even use it for curls. We recommend titanium plates, like the ones we use in the Drybar Tress Press. They heat up fast and evenly, and straighten hair in one go. Look for an iron that has a slightly beveled rather than blunt edge, so you can give your ends a bit of movement.

Nozzles

Nozzles are attachments that help direct air flow. There are two types of nozzles: A smaller, more narrow nozzle that gives max concentration of heat and air, making it handy when smoothing out highly textured, or coarse and curly hair, and a larger nozzle that gives you a wider dispersion of air. Since the width of the larger nozzle is typically close to the length of the brush, it makes it ideal for creating curls. Nozzles are optional (and we don't even like to use them when we are rough drying hair!).

Our "High Tops" self grip rollers come in two sizes

Self-Grip Rollers

When you want big hair and want to avoid that awesome bed-head split (aka cat butt), sleeping in a few self-grip rollers will do the trick. You can also use them to help build volume while styling your hair. They're most effective when set in warm hair, and as it cools they hold the shape and create volume. By no means are these as crucial to styling as, say, a blow-dryer, but they make me happy and I think they'll make you happy too.

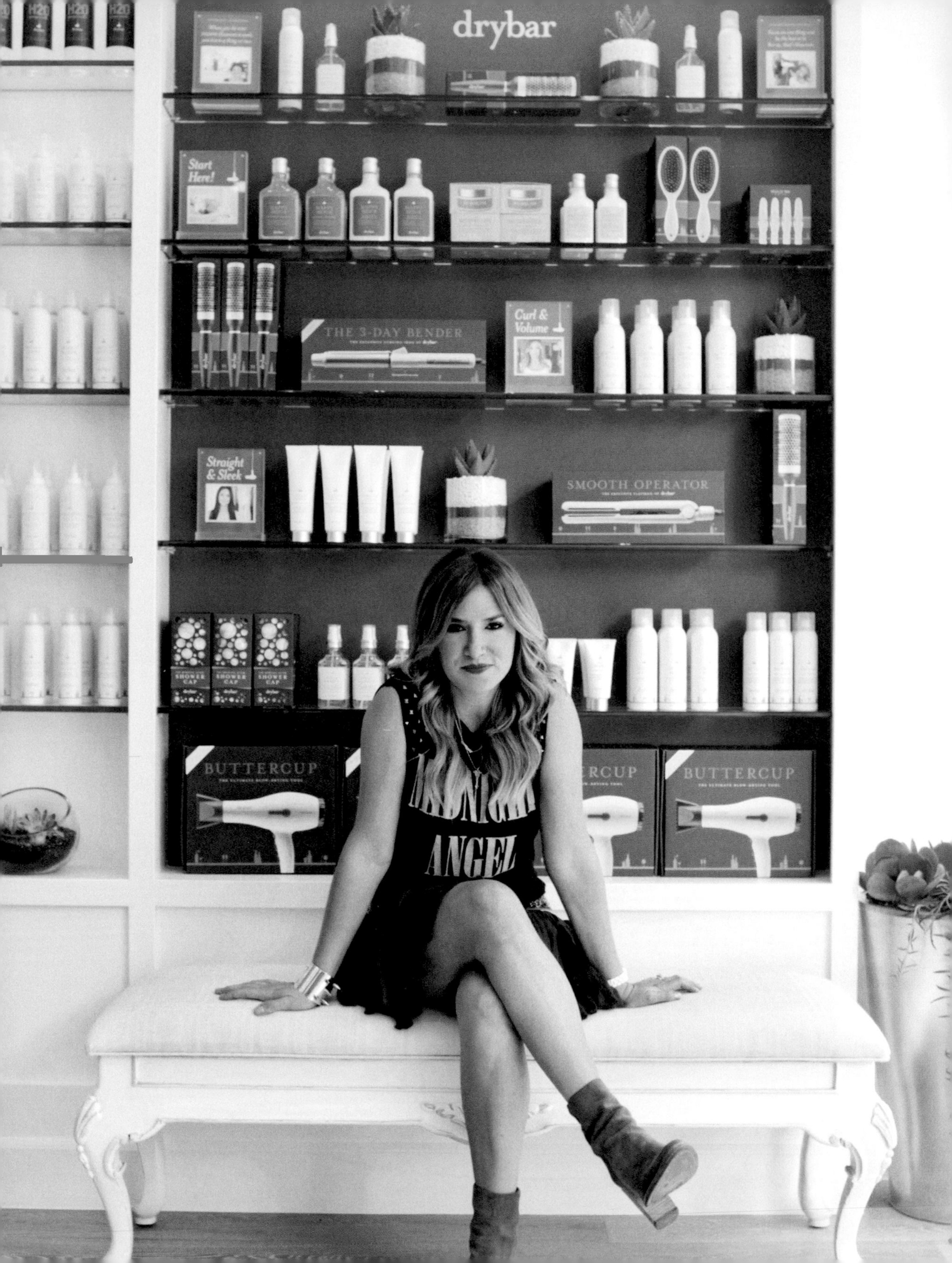
drybar
Start Here!
THE 3-DAY BENDER
Curl & Volume
Straight & Sleek
SMOOTH OPERATOR
SHOWER CAP
BUTTERCUP
ANGEL

PRODUCTS

Shampoo

A great blowout starts with really clean hair! Dirty, oily hair never blows out well, and the style won't last as long as it should. Shampoo should remove buildup without stripping your hair of its natural oils and drying it out. If your hair is baby-fine, look for a gentle cleansing shampoo. For dry hair, look for formulas that are labeled hydrating or moisturizing, and nourish the hair from the inside out.

Conditioner

It seems simple enough, but finding the right conditioner for your hair is a game changer. Many women make the mistake of choosing a conditioner that is too heavy and wind up with hair that's weighed down. Think about your hair type and then make your choice: For fine hair or hair that tends to feel oily quickly, you'll want something light but hydrating, and focus on the ends, avoiding the roots; for dry hair, choose a deep conditioner that will give it that extra love and hydration. Anyone with extra-dry hair or hair that tangles easily could benefit big-time from a few spritzes of leave-in conditioner and a biweekly mask or treatment.

Heat Protectant

This is your insurance policy against damage. After towel-drying and before styling, applying heat protectant all over helps seal split ends and prevents dryness, damage, and breakage—and a really good one, like our Hot Toddy, also shields hair from UV exposure, which can zap the life out of color-treated hair. It's like your seat belt, bike helmet, and Stay Puft Marshmallow Man suit all in one. Everyone should use it.

Hydrating Cream

It's just what your tough locks have been waiting for. Medium to coarse hair reaps the most benefit from a hydrating cream, since the right formula will deliver needed moisture, smooth the cuticle, and protect your hair from the heat.

Volumizer

Depending on your hair type, you'll want to pump up the volume with a mousse or a spray. Either way, volumizers

Opening day of
Drybar Encino, CA
Summer 2013

help build body by coating each strand of hair, making for a fuller look with more movement.

Shine Cream

When hair is dry, it can look dull. A shine cream will brighten it right up. It will calm flyaways near the roots and bring thirsty-looking ends back to life. Look for a product that also moisturizes—no crispy pieces, please.

Shine Spray

Lightly misting dry hair with a shine spray will help tame static and frizz, and leave it looking glossy, as the name implies. Most formulas contain oils that hydrate hair and help reflect light.

Hair Spray

A good hair spray will add some shine and keep your style in place without turning it into a helmet. You want to be able to reapply the spray as needed without it building up, flaking off, or getting sticky. And you should definitely be able to run a brush through your hair at the end of the night.

Paste

Without hair paste, there would be no Justin Bieber. This is the stuff that makes boy bands' worlds go round. A workable paste will create texture, definition, and hold. It can be the secret ingredient in polished-looking up-dos, ponytails, and braids, and work wonders on hiding baby hairs around the face.

Hair Oil

Dry and damaged hair loves this stuff. I'm talking loves. Hair oil replenishes much-needed hydration especially to coarse and curly hair, or to particularly sad strands. When using hair oil, concentrate on the ends. Get too close to the crown and things can start looking very greasy, very quickly.

Dry Shampoo

It's a blowout's best friend. Adding a bit of powder to your roots soaks up excess oils and impurities and creates texture and lift. I never leave home without it (neither should you).

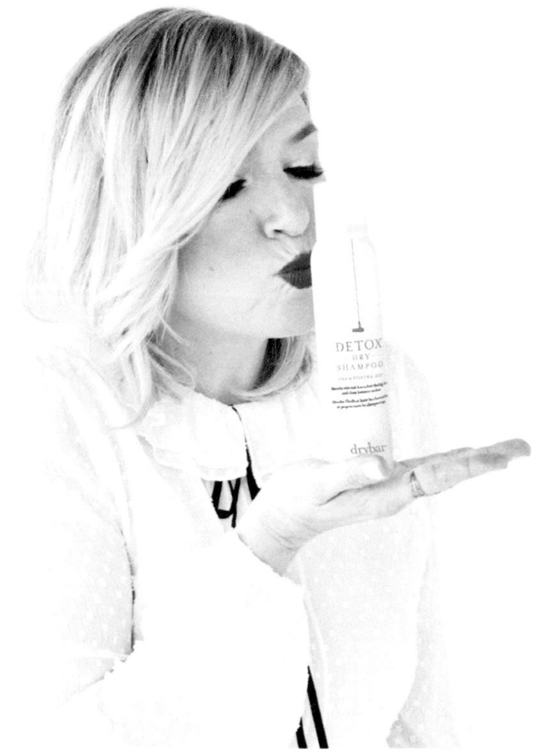

Dry Conditioner
This is like a refresh button for your hair. While dry shampoo works its magic on the scalp, dry conditioner takes care of everything else from midshaft to ends, adding a silky shine and major hydration for dry, crispy ends.

Silk Pillowcase
Smooth silk fibers, unlike the more textured cotton or linen in standard pillowcases, help keep cuticles nice and smooth and prevent epic bed head.

Shower Cap
Your grandma was a smart lady. A shower cap is the very best way to protect your blowout from moisture when you're in the shower (or even taking a bath!).

SHOP TALK: HOW TO SOUND LIKE A PRO

Don't know your hair shaft from your elbow? Here's a quick overview of the most important hairstyling terms (and some things we just say all the time!) to know and love.

Antennae: The baby hairs that sprout up right at your hairline or along your part. We are constantly trying to calm these down. The secret: Don't use too much tension on them when they are wet. Rough-dry the fringe to calm them down.

Body: When we use the word body, we're referring to the fullness throughout your hair. Some people like a lot of body and bounce, others prefer zero-body for a pin-straight look.

Breakage: The tell-tale signs of breakage are frayed ends, uneven length, and a lot of hair left in the brush. When hair just can't take it anymore, it just. Breaks. Off. Overstyling or overprocessing your hair, plus lack of moisture, is often the culprit, but the health of your hair is also directly connected to diet, stress, and illness. Eat healthy, take care of yourself, and make time for hair treatments and masks.

Frizz: In a word: annoying. When the cuticle of your hair is lifted, moisture poofs up the strand, making it appear rough instead of smooth.

Midshaft: The middle point of the length of your hair. Of course, this is different on everyone, so in relation to styling, brushes, and hot tools, the midshaft starts 4 to 6 inches (10 to 14 cm) away from the scalp.

Overdirection: Essential to building volume (mostly at the root) and giving the hair life, this technique takes hair up and over the head rather than straight out or down.

Part: The line where hair is divided. Pretty simple. It can be down the center, off to the side, way down deep on the side, or at an angle. Whether it's where your hair naturally falls or you set it with a comb, a part is a part.

Roots: While each hair has a root of its own, when stylists talk about roots and say things like "at the root" or "from roots to ends," they are referring to the hair right at the scalp.

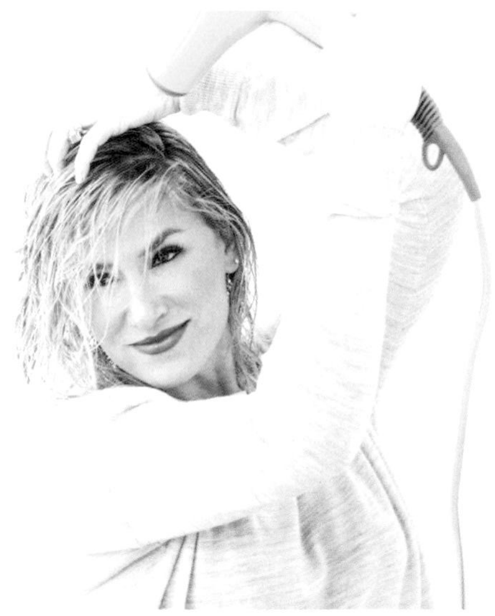

Rough-Drying: Taking the moisture out of your hair with just the blow-dryer and your fingers before you start working your sections with a brush.

Section: This is a clearly defined area of your hair. You'll hear a lot about sectioning, which refers to cleanly dividing the hair into zones, and subsectioning, which is dividing a section into smaller, more manageable pieces.

Texture: The look, feel, condition, and consistency of each strand of hair define your hair texture. Smooth and thick, wavy and fine, curly and dry, the combinations are endless.

Volume: The term we use for the amount of lift, especially at the root. Other terms we might throw around: height, lift, boost, oomph, va-va-voom.

SECTION 3:

HEY, GOOD LOOKIN'

Drybar's Signature Styles

When I first started daydreaming about Drybar, I would constantly come up with ways to fix the little (and big) things that got on people's nerves when they went into a traditional salon. Everyone seemed to complain about the language barrier between stylists and clients. The client says, "Just a trim." The stylist says, "I'll just take the ends off." And in the end, someone is left crying about her new bob. I want to live in a world where a soft curl means a soft curl and a loose wave means exactly that (don't we all?).

And that's how our menu came about. After narrowing down the millions of possibilities to the most in-demand and timeless styles, we named each one after a cocktail, snapped photos to show them off, and created our first lookbooks for the shop. This way, women could just point at what they wanted, their stylist could give them exactly what they were after, and everyone lived happily ever after. What could be easier than that?

Now, before we get started on teaching you how to do these looks at home, it's time to go over the Drybar Buttercup Code. Everyone's hair may be crazily different, but whatever style you're going for, the best results come from sticking to a few simple rules. These tried-and-true tips will set you up for maximum success whether your hair is short or long, straight or curly, picture-perfect or no-photos-please.

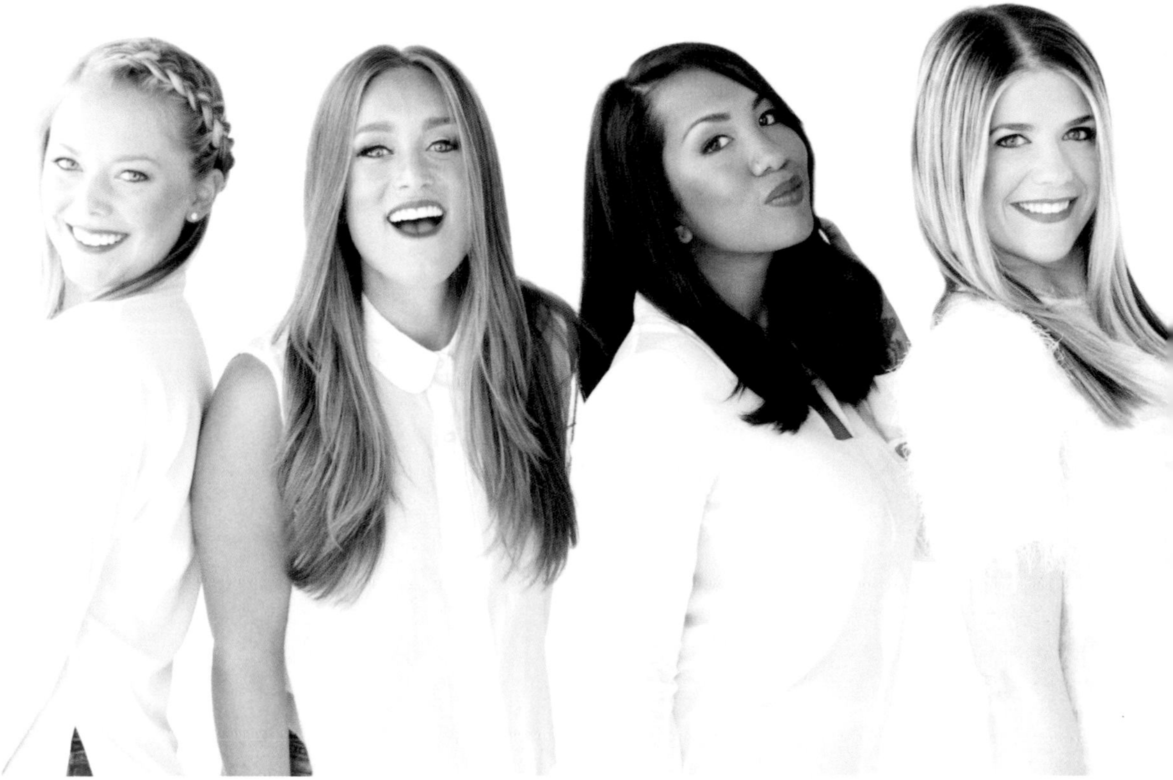

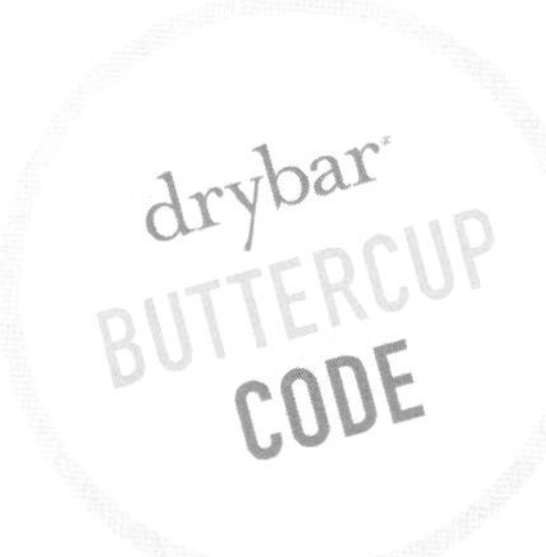

1. **Make a Clean Start**
   I've said it before and I'll say it again, one trillion times or more: Squeaky-clean and well-conditioned hair is the foundation of a good blowout. Running your hair under the faucet or spraying your whole head down does not count. Dirt, oil, residue from products, and environmental buildup just complicate things and compromise your style—and ruin any chances for any bounce. Boo, who wants that?

2. **Towel-Dry before Blow-Dry**
   Getting rid of excess moisture won't only speed up the blow-dry process; it will also allow the products you do use to be absorbed better, so you'll get the most out of them. (Don't brush your hair yet!)

3. **Always Use Protection**
   And this means applying heat protectant all over, roots to ends. It will help lock in hydration, prevent breakage, and keep hair healthy. This is especially important if you get blowouts (of course you do, or why would you be reading this book?!) or often use heat to style your hair (I mean, who doesn't?). You wouldn't bake on the beach without sunscreen on, would you? (And if you said yes, who are you? Me in 1995?) (Don't brush it yet!)

4. **Go Easy on the Good Stuff**
   When you're using the right products, a little should go a long way. Volumizing products like mousses and sprays are really the only styling products that should get anywhere near your root, capisce? For most everything else that goes on pre-blow-dry, start with a small amount in the palm of your hand, rub palms together, and apply from midshaft to ends. You can always use more if you need to. If your hair starts to feel greasy, flat, or heavy, that's a sign you've used too much! (Still don't brush it!)

5. **Get Even**
   Always distribute product evenly by working it through your hair with a wide-tooth comb or a detangling brush. Start at the bottom and work your way up to make sure you get out all the knots (and don't make them worse). Running your fingers through your hair or smooshing product into your ends is cheating, and you'll be able to tell when you get crunchy bits or a section that just won't behave.

6. **Own the VIP Section**
   Very. Important. Parting. Sectioning is the road map of your hair style. Since every style is different, refer to the step-by-step for exact instructions, but this is generally how it's going to go:

   - Set your part. Your hair dries the way you let it lie, so even if you're air-drying, draw your part in while your hair is still damp.

- Draw on a headband; always work from ear to ear, forward. Twist the rest of your hair in the back into a bun and clip to stay put and damp.
- Begin with your bangs. They usually have a tricky cowlick that needs immediate attention and they're what people see first on you—so make 'em look good. Work the front in vertical subsections from ear to ear.
- When you are ready to dry the back, draw a horizontal line from the back of one ear to the back of the other to create top and bottom sections. Twist and clip up the top. Divide the lower section into two, twist and clip one section aside, and work in subsections from ear to ear. Push sections of dry hair forward, in front of your shoulders, to keep it as far away from the wet sections as possible. (Avoid putting wet hair on dry hair, eek!)
- Divide the top section into two, and work in subsections until all your hair is dry.

7. **Have Fun!**
   This is our mantra at Drybar for both our clients and our stylists. Life's too short to have it any other way, right? So if you can't make it to a Drybar (aw, we will be thinking of you), set your own mood with a little good lighting, an awesome playlist, funny movies, something fizzy in a fancy flute—or even just a slice of lemon in a glass of water; it can all do wonders for your mood. Definitely try this at home.

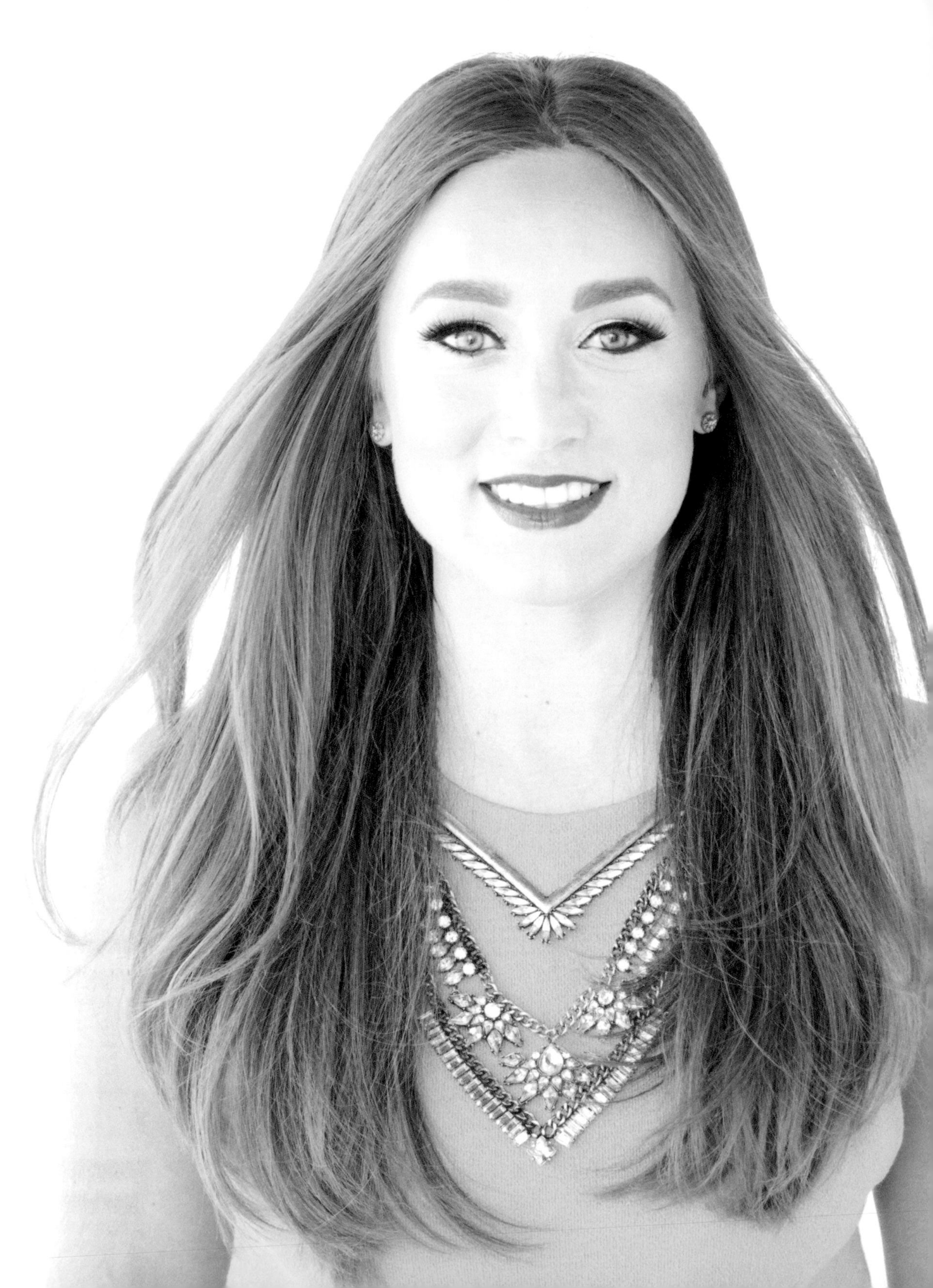

– THE –

STRAIGHT UP

STRAIGHT WITH A LITTLE BIT OF BODY

LIGHT AND BREEZY NICE AND EASY

Ingredients:

Leave-in conditioner

Hydrating control cream (for my curly/coarse/frizzy ladies)

Mousse (for the fine/straight manes)

Detangling brush

Clips

Blow-dryer

Nozzle

Medium round ceramic-barrel brush

Large barrel curling iron

Shine cream

Flexible-hold hair spray

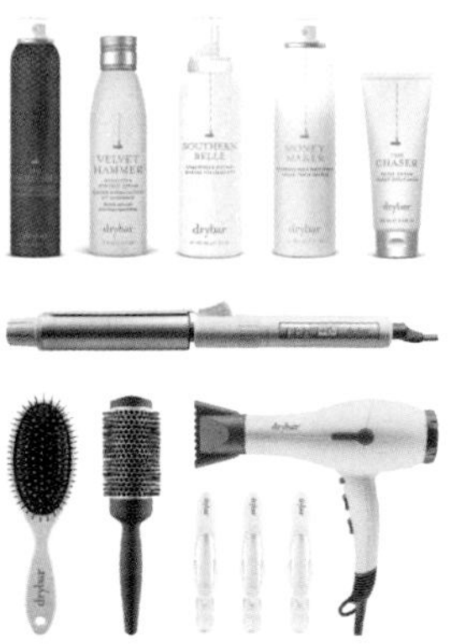

Allow me to introduce the Straight Up. It just so happens to be one of my personal favorites, but that's not why it's the first style in this book. It's really the building block of all blowouts: Whether you have straightish hair or your hair is coarse and curly, the end result is pretty and polished.

It's also one of the most versatile styles that can really last: A little dry shampoo and a curling iron can give it a whole new look. In fact, I start most Mondays with a Straight Up, and by Wednesday, I'm ready for a Mai Tai or messy Cosmo to help me cruise through the rest of the workweek.

The most important thing to remember about this style is to take your time. This isn't the kind of style to be rushed through. It takes patience to make sure that you cover every section thoroughly, and a bit of practice to make sure you leave the ends bouncy and soft.

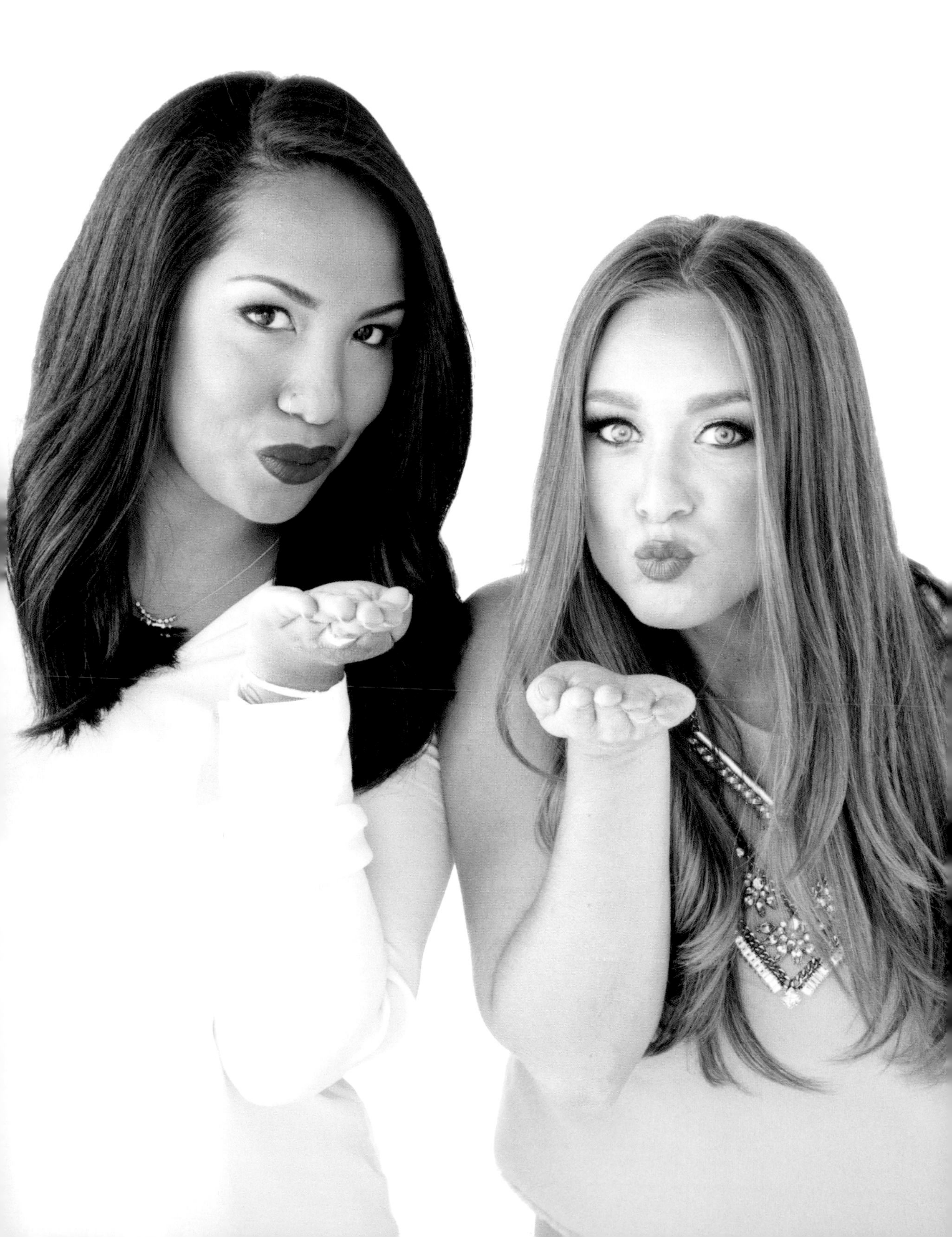

1. Naturally coarse hair needs a little extra love, so mastering the right combination of products, tools, and tension while blow drying is key.

2. After washing and conditioning, towel dry your hair.

For very **textured** hair: Spray a leave-in conditioner like Mr. Incredible from midshaft to ends. Follow with a hydrating control cream like Velvet Hammer, also applied from midshaft to ends. Always keep cream and oil-based products away from your roots.

For hair that's naturally **straight**, build body by adding a volumizing mousse like Southern Belle. Rub a generous dollop between your palms and apply to damp hair from roots to ends. Brush through hair to distribute evenly.

3. Spray a leave-in conditioner like Mr. Incredible all over, then follow with a hydrating control cream like Velvet Hammer throughout. If your hair is fine or gets oily easily, apply product from midshaft to ends. And keep cream and oil-based products away from your roots.

4. Set your part to road-map your style. Brush product through hair to distribute evenly.

1

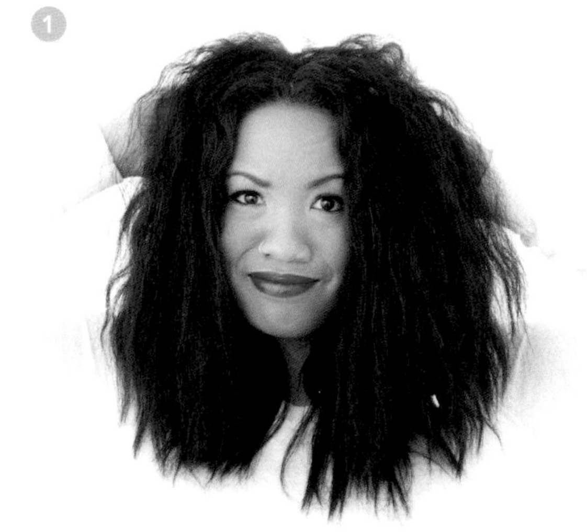

4

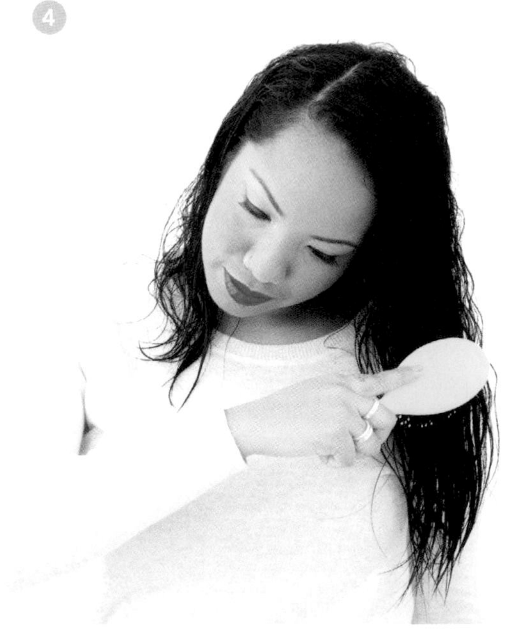

2

3

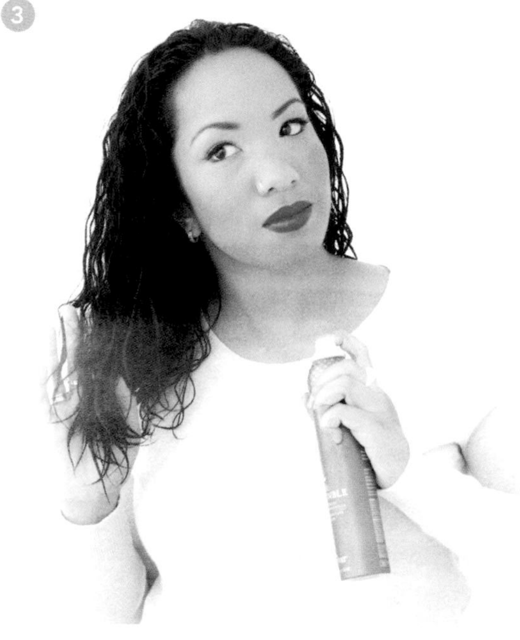

5

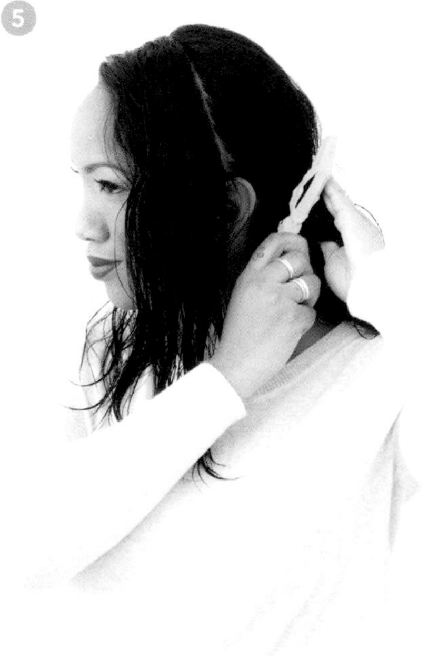

5. Section hair from ear to ear. Secure the back with a clip. Keep damp hair clipped tight to help hold in the moisture until you get around to blow-drying the crown and back sections.

6. Pop a nozzle onto your blow-dryer. Working in vertical subsections, scoop hair up at the roots with a ceramic-barrel brush like the Full Pint, and roll from roots to ends away from the face. Repeat, repeat, repeat!

For **longer hair**, just use a round ceramic brush with a bigger barrel. For extreme curls and textured roots, use a boar-bristle brush instead!

7. As you dry each section, be sure to roll the brush through to the very end for a smooth, bouncy blowout.

8. Continue to work vertical subsections on the other side. Make sure each section is completely dry before moving on, but do your best to work in quick, short bursts.

9. Section out the back of the hair in to three sections; bottom, middle and crown. Start blowdrying the hair at the nape and making sure to point the blow dryer down the hair shaft.

10. As you work up the head, roll hair in and out, and release with a twist of the wrist to create a bit of movement. Continue to work similar sections up to the crown of the head.

11. To build volume at the crown, blow-dry horizontal sections straight up and back, away from the face. You can also set this section in a self-grip roller like a High Top for even more volume; allow to set (while you get dressed or put on makeup). The longer it cools and sets, the more volume you'll have.

6

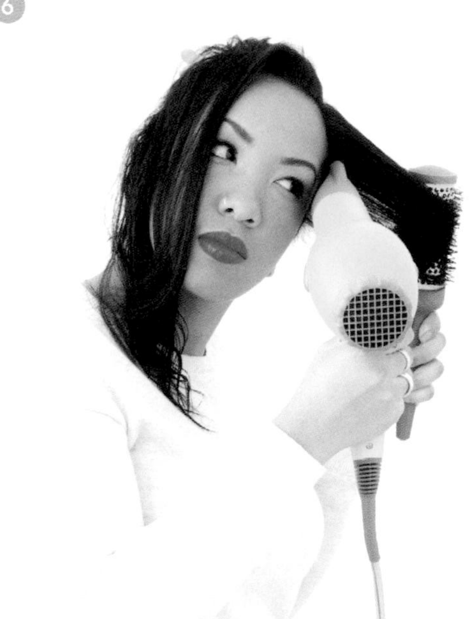

9

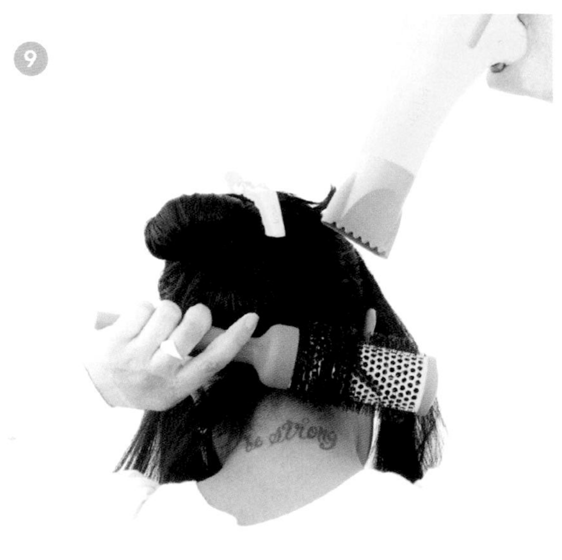

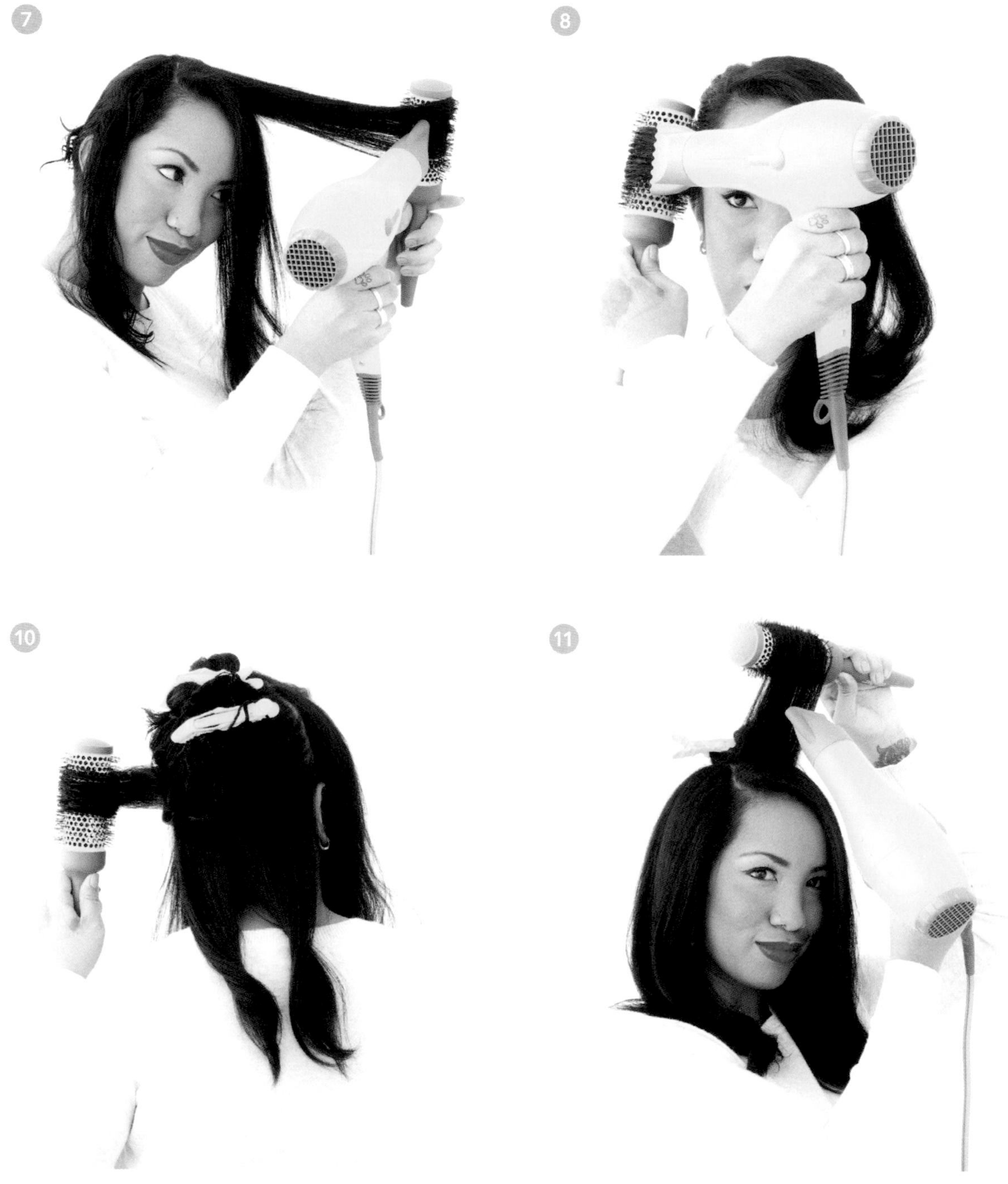
7
8
10
11

12

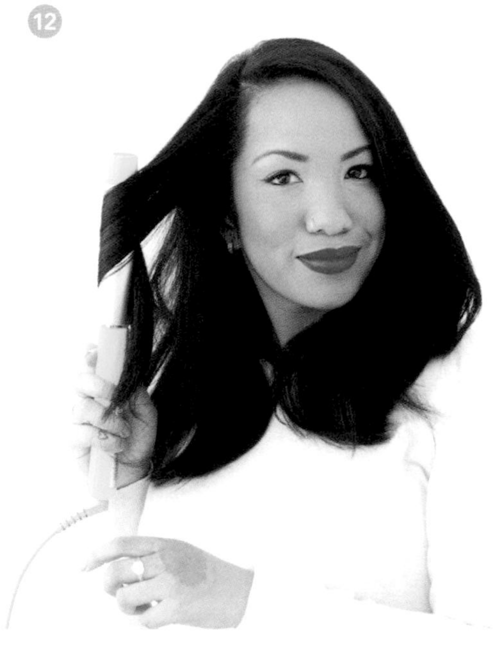

13

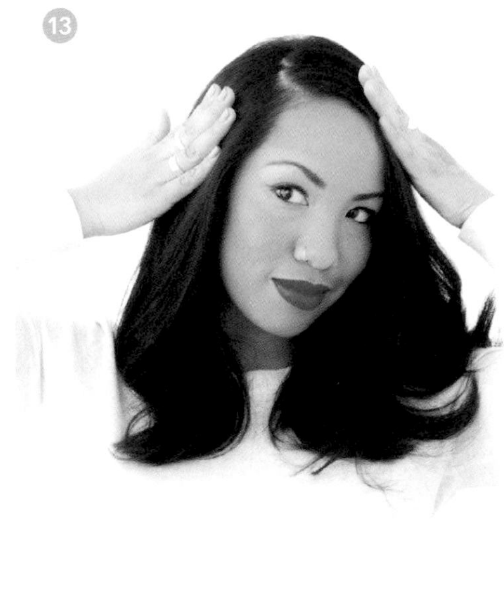

14

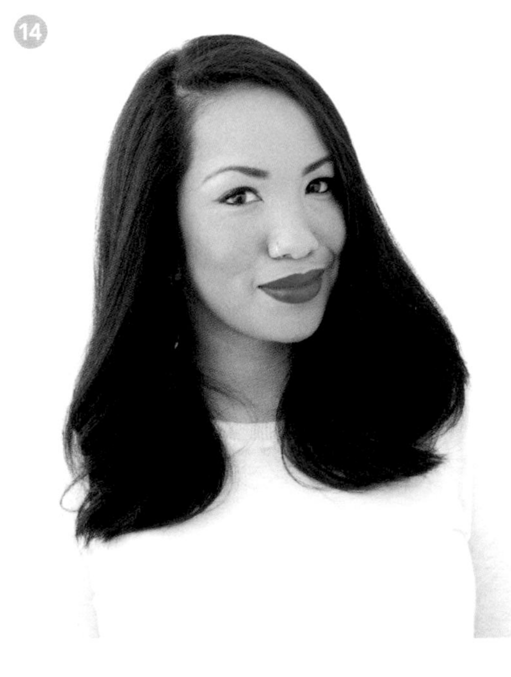

12. To polish your look and get rid of any frizz, wrap wide vertical sections of hair around a larger barrel of a preheated curling iron like the 3-Day Bender. Hold just for a couple of seconds and barely give it a twist. This is mainly for smoothing and locking in the shape you created during the blowout.

13. Finish with a shine cream like the Chaser. Rub a pea-size amount of product between your palms. Using your fingers, rake softly through your hair, being careful not to mat it down.

14. For extra shine and hold, spray all over with a light mist of flexible-hold hair spray like Money Maker.

WE LIKE TO THINK THE STRAIGHT UP

IS FOR A NO-NONSENSE TYPE OF LADY

WHO KNOWS EXACTLY WHAT SHE WANTS.

IT CAN EASILY MORPH INTO A COSMO OR A MAI TAI.

IT'S ALSO ONE OF THE EASIEST TO ACHIEVE

AND ONCE YOU GET THIS ONE DOWN,

ALL THE OTHER STYLES WILL FALL IN LINE.

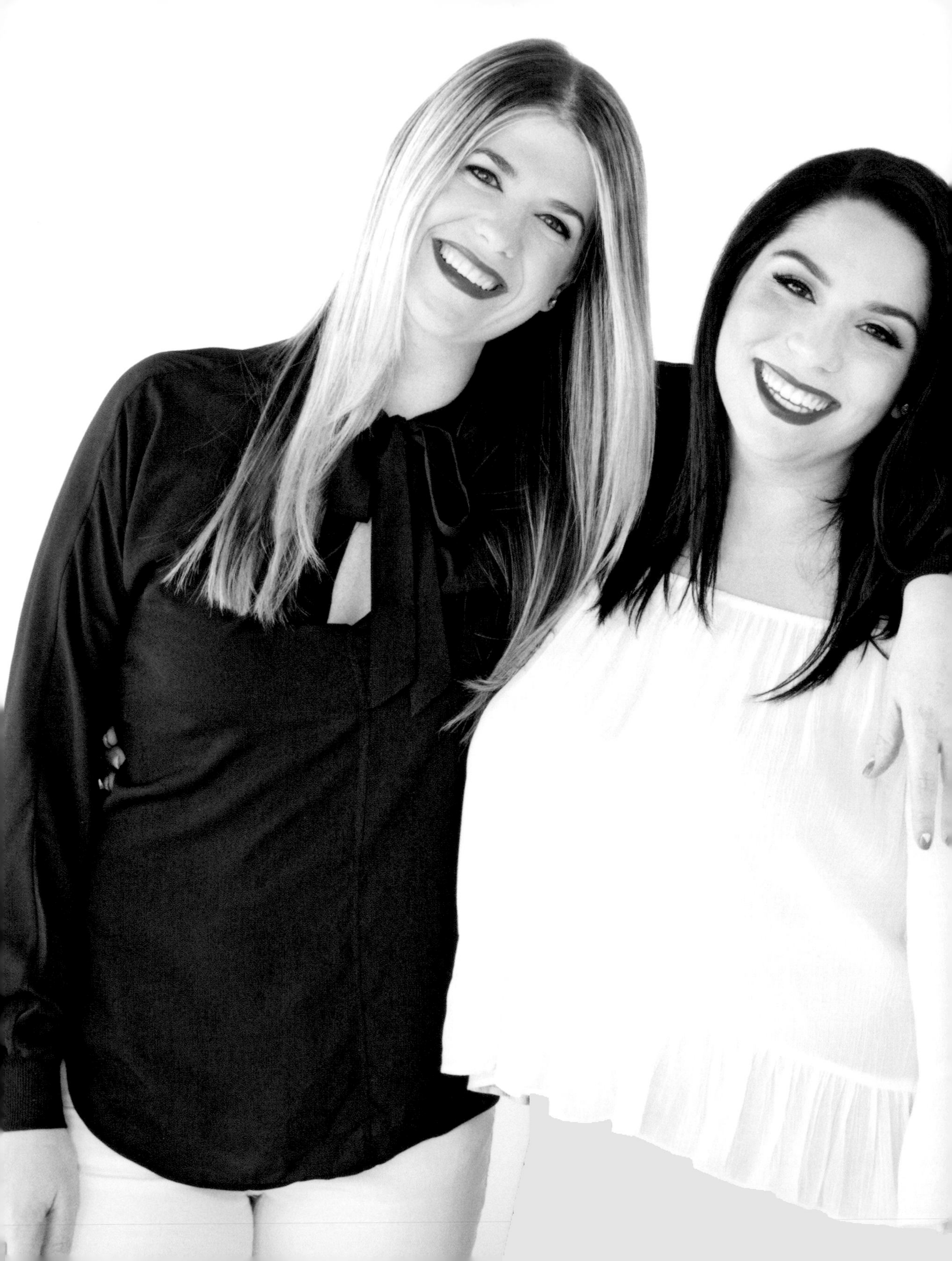

- THE -
MANHATTAN

SLEEK AND SMOOTH

THE MANHATTAN

WORK IT

Ingredients:

Heat protectant

Hydrating control cream

Detangling brush

Clips

Medium round ceramic-barrel brush

Large round ceramic-barrel brush

Blow-dryer

Nozzle

Flat iron

Flexible-hold hair spray

Hair oil

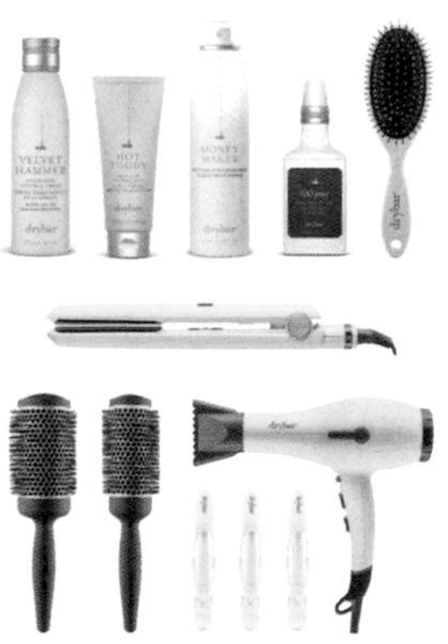

The Manhattan is the power style that looks just like it sounds: seriously straight, maxed-out shine, and a zero-tolerance policy in the frizz department.

Ladies with fine, straight hair, you could make this look happen in two secs–it might even be what happens when you part, comb through, and let your hair air-dry. But if this is what your hair does when it's left to its own devices, you're probably not interested in doing it this way at home.

That said, all my textured, wavy, and medium/coarse-haired girls, follow along. After getting your hair nice, smooth, and straight during the blowout, you may want to use a flat iron to zap any static, seal the ends and up the shine. Remember to plug in your flat iron so it's ready when you are. Using an iron while the temperature is in flux could cause you to overwork a section and give you inconsistent results. I like to use the flat iron to finish the ends with the slightest bit of bend.

1. This is what we call medium, wavy, frizzy hair. A little bit of everything! And that volume is real, thanks to the curl that comes in at the roots.

2. After towel-drying, apply a heat protectant like Hot Toddy all over, and follow with a hydrating control cream like Velvet Hammer from midshaft to ends. Brush through. Pop a nozzle on your dryer. Part and section hair. Now, rough-dry your hair, keeping the air flow downward.

If your hair is **super fine** and a little **unruly**, after towel-drying, apply a lightweight smoothing cream like the Chaser on the ends. That's about all you'll need.

3. Starting in the front, subsection out the baby hair and shorter pieces framing the face into as many sections as you would like. It's going to take some heat and a lot of tension to smooth out the curl.

4. Using a medium round ceramic-barrel brush (you can also use a boar-bristle brush at a very curly hairline), pick up hair from behind the section at the roots, and use lots of tension as you roll the brush through to the ends. Keep the nozzle of the dryer very close to the brush. Don't be afraid to really get in there. Repeat, repeat, repeat!

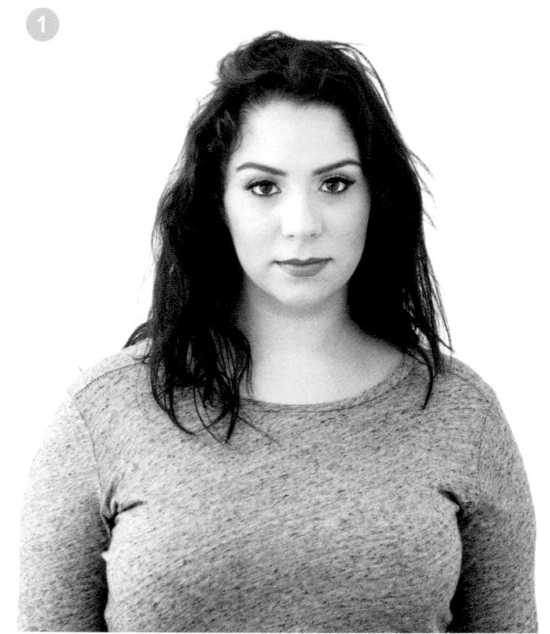

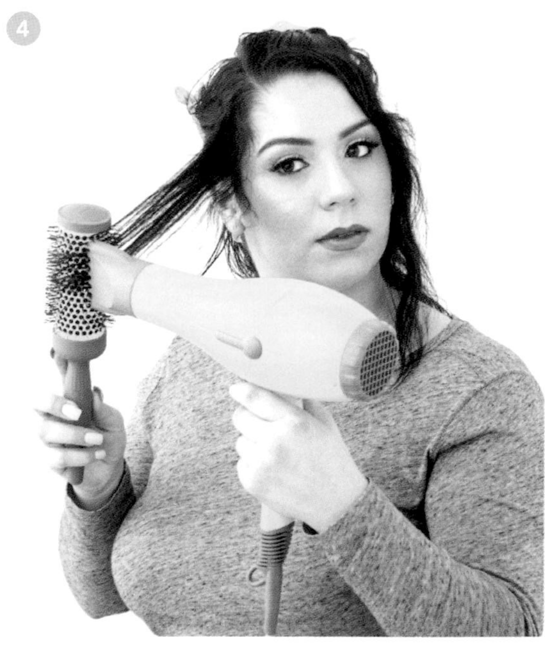

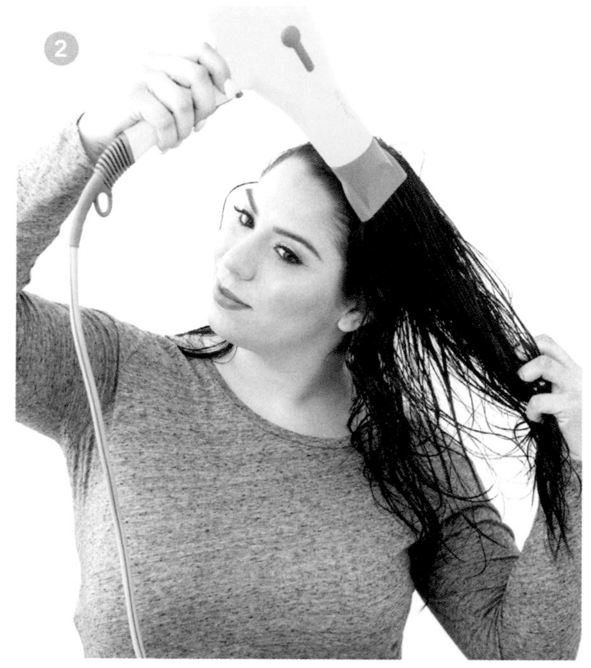

2

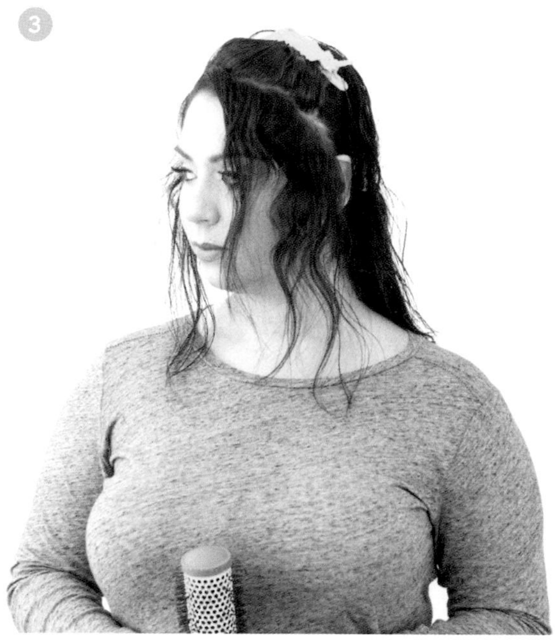

3

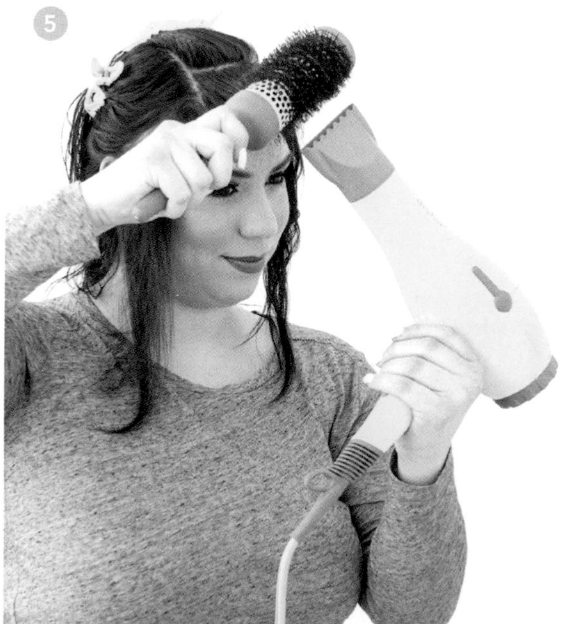

5

5. Starting from your part, pick up a horizontal section from your hairline and blow forward and up, rolling from roots to ends.

Short Cut for Short Bangs: To avoid the dreaded 1980s puffy **bangs**, blow-dry bangs and roll the brush away from your face and down, sweeping them across your forehead in both directions.

6. Blend the front and side sections together. Pick up hair from behind and roll the brush from roots to ends, angling down and away. Focus a little longer on the ends to give them a slight bend—not a full curl.

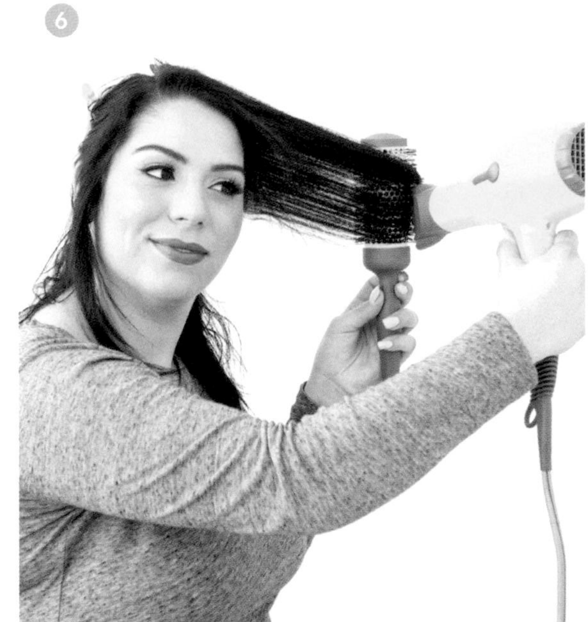

7. To dry the back of your hair, you'll divide this area into three parts. First, draw a horizontal line to create a small section at the nape of the neck. Twist and clip the rest of your hair at the crown.

8. Using a large round ceramic-barrel brush, pick up hair at the roots so the hair lies on top of the brush, and roll from roots to ends as you dry. Always work in manageable subsections. It's OK if they are small—you run into trouble when sections are too big.

9. Keep working up toward the crown, making sure to twist and clip the wet hair out of your way. Drop down horizontal sections as you go, using as much tension as possible. Now's a great time to plug in a flat iron like the Tress Press.

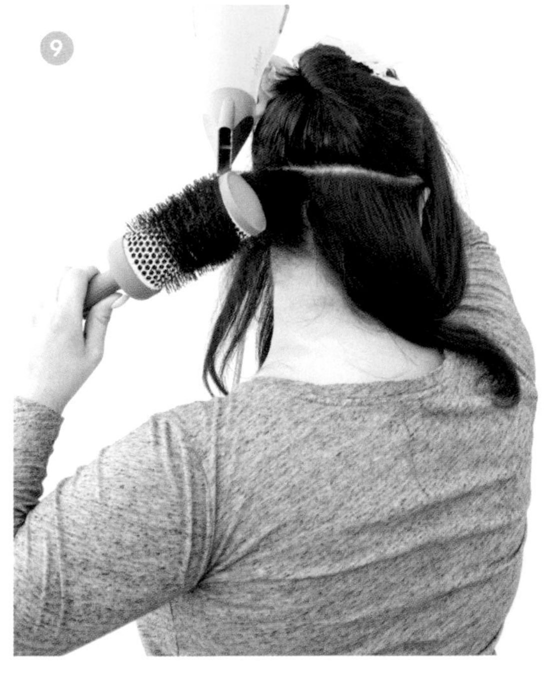

10. To dry the crown, work in horizontal sections, starting with the brush underneath the hair, and roll the brush from roots to ends, pulling the hair up and slightly forward using lots of tension. This will give you just the right amount of lift.

11. Now that the blowout is complete, get ready to start flatironing. One pass of the iron should do the trick, but don't be afraid to go back over your hair again quickly if it is textured or coarse.

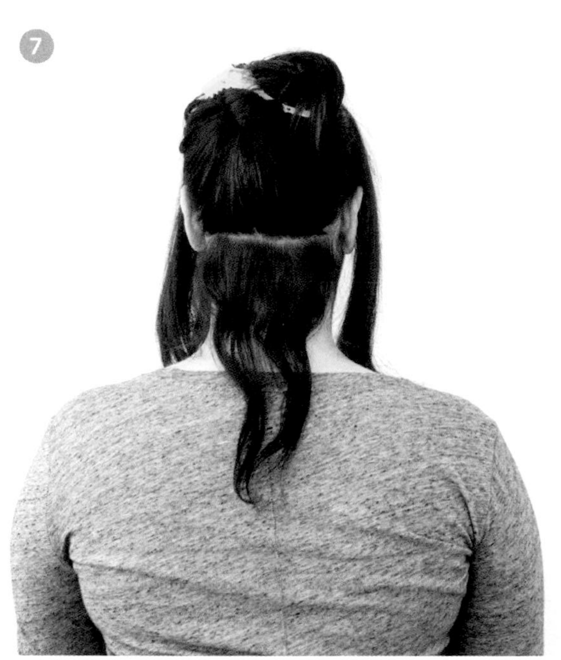
7

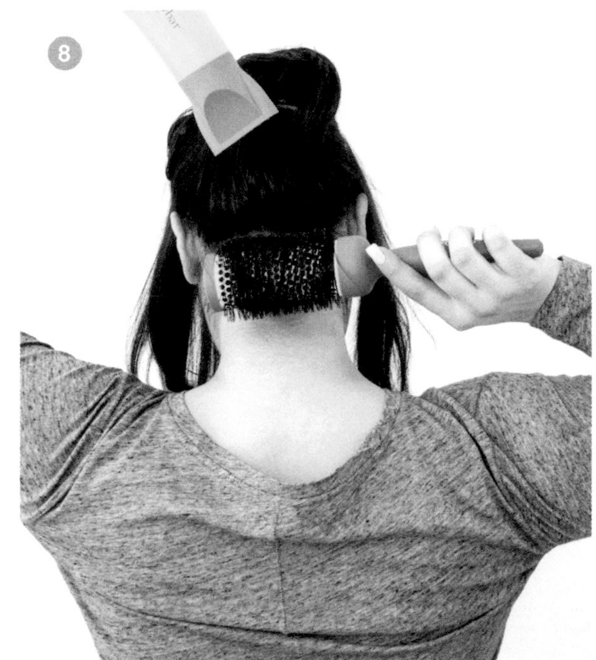
8

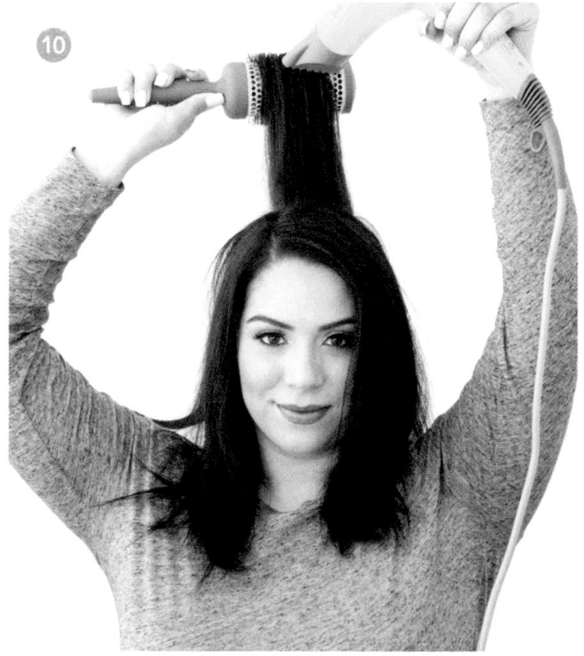
10

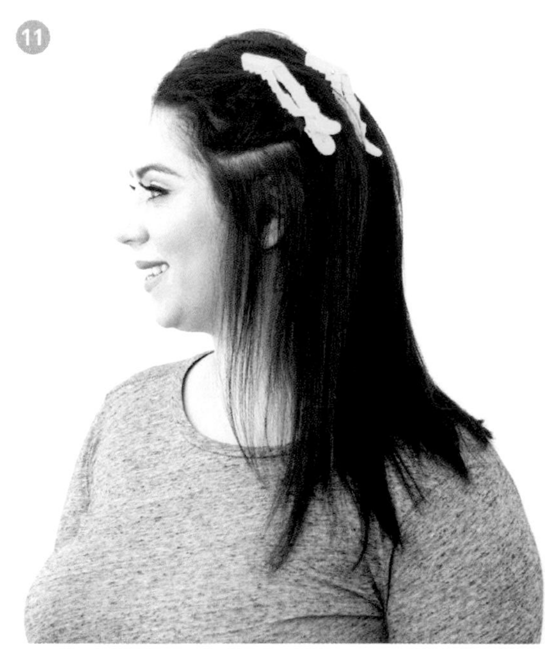
11

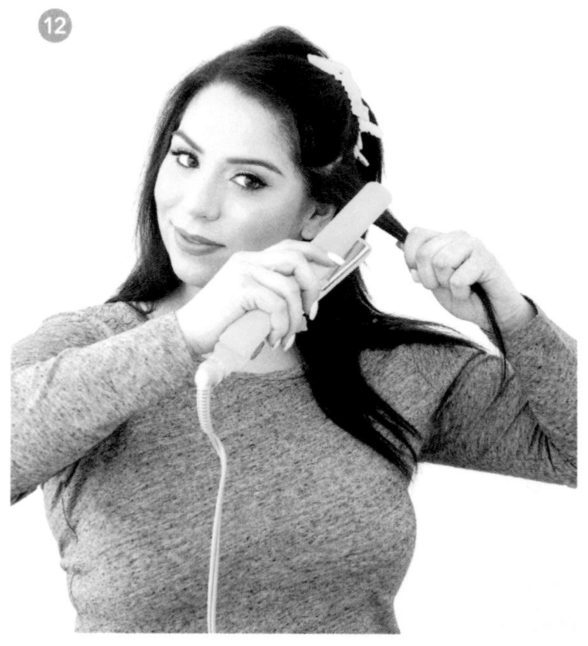

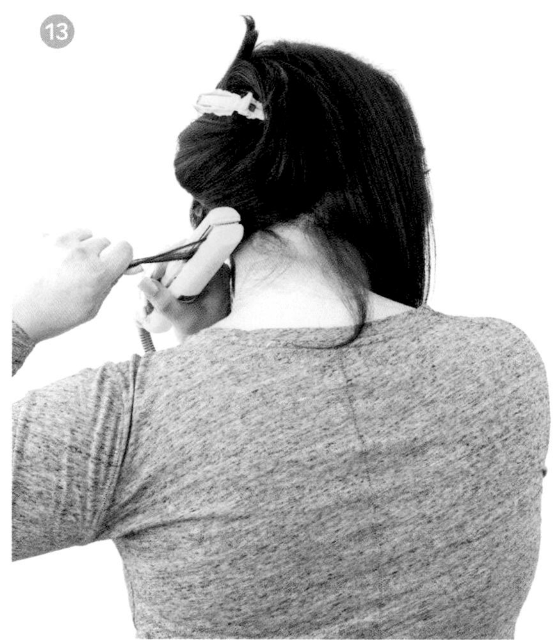

12. With each subsection of hair, draw the iron down from roots to ends, beveling the ends just barely. The tiniest bit of flick gives this super straight style more movement, for a less severe look.

13. Start with the iron close to the roots to smooth any frizz or leftover wave.

14. Spray with a flexible hold hair spray like Money Maker to help set and keep hair super smooth. For any antennae or flyaways at your part, spray just a burst or two of hair spray into your hand, rub palms together, and pat hairs down using a light touch. Lastly, add a little touch of treatment oil like 100 Proof to seal the ends.

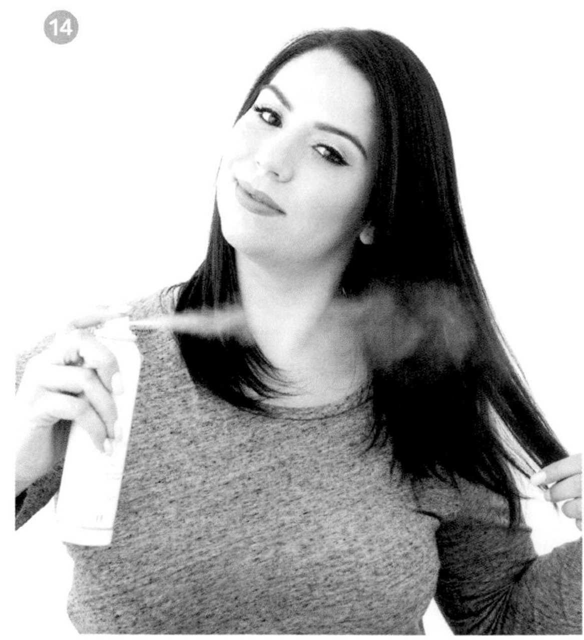

POWER WOMAN!

THIS STRAIGHT AND SLEEK LOOK
MAKES YOU FEEL VERY IN CONTROL
AND LIKE YOU CAN TAKE ON THE WORLD.
NOT TO MENTION, WHEN THIS
LOOK IS PROPERLY EXECUTED,
YOUR HAIR LOOKS LIKE SILK.

IT'S A TOTAL WIN-WIN.

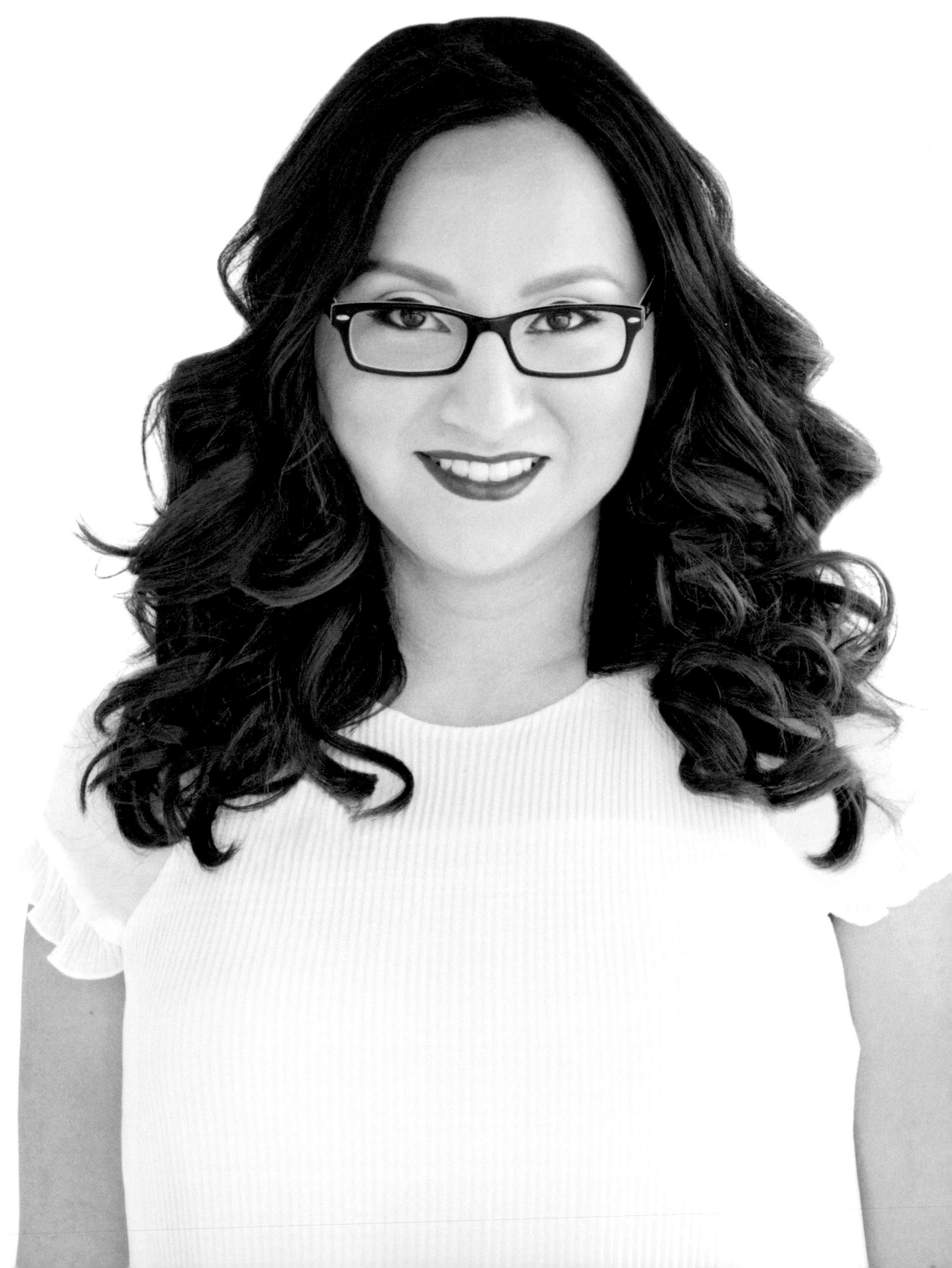

- THE -

COSMO

LOTS OF LOOSE CURLS

THE COSMO

THE PARTY'S OVER HERE

Ingredients:

Volumizing mousse

Heat protectant

Detangling brush

Clips

Small round ceramic-barrel brush (for shorter hair)

Medium round ceramic-barrel brush (for longer hair)

Blow-dryer

Medium barrel curling iron (for shorter hair)

Large barrel curling iron (for longer hair)

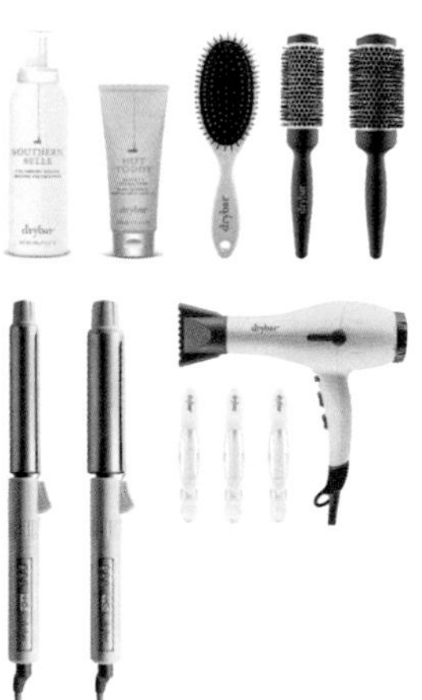

The Manhattan may be your Monday-morning, coffee-at-your-desk, ready-to-tackle-that-overflowing-email-inbox hairstyle, which makes the Cosmo your Saturday night.

Whether you're feeling blah about your look or about your life, the Cosmo is a foolproof pick-me-up. Fine, straight hair will need products that will build texture to help hold the curl, plus extra love from the curling iron. Getting hair with a natural wave to play the curl factor up should be a cinch—just make sure to finish with shine cream or shine serum and hair spray to keep flyaways out of sight.

This style is all about bouncy curls, tousled just so, making it both polished and pretty and also fun and flirty.

The Cosmo is a real good time.

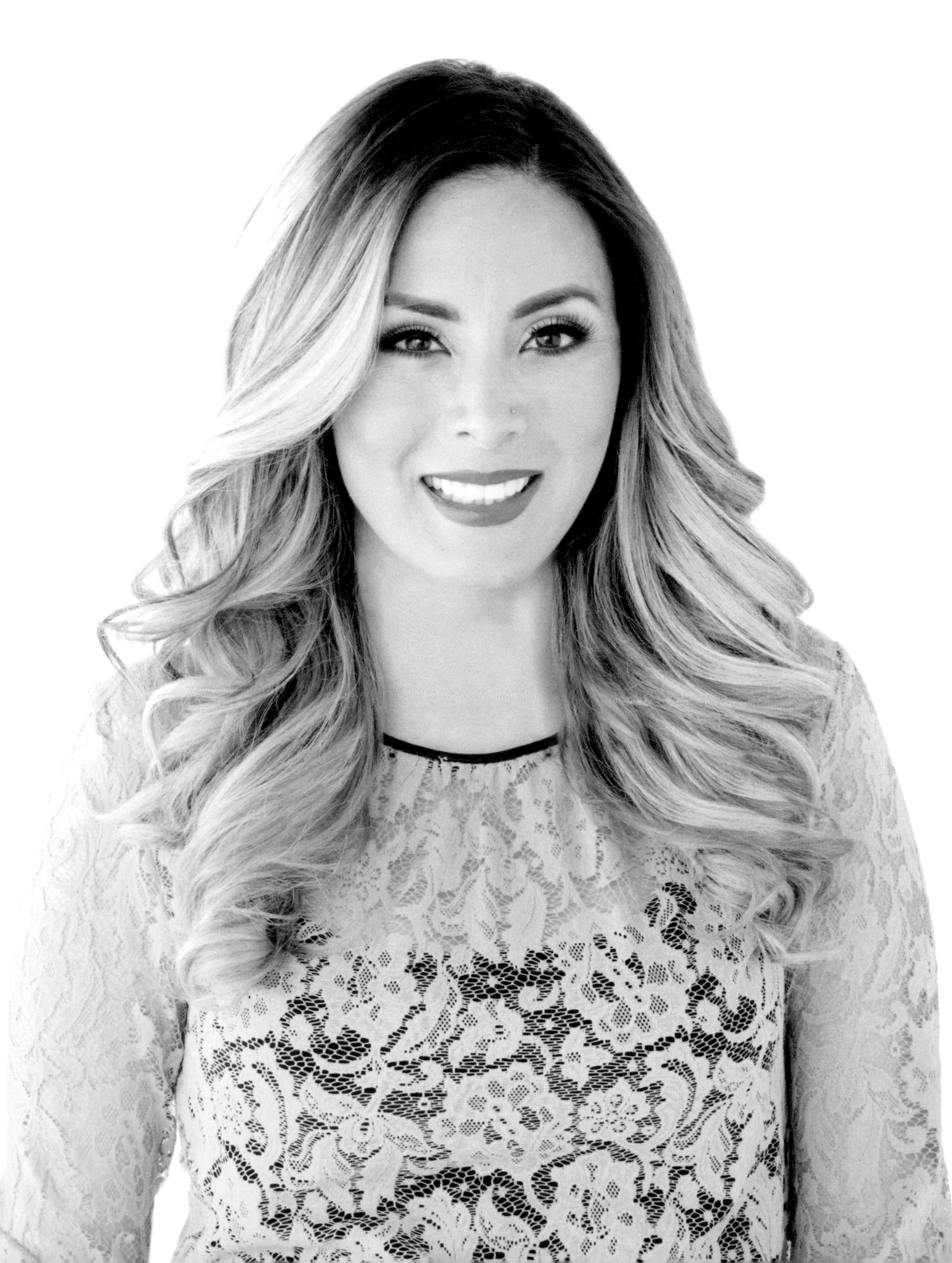

1. This is what it looks like when you have naturally frizzy, fine hair, but lots of it. In other words, like, whoa, help! After washing, conditioning, and towel-drying your hair, apply a volumizing mousse like Southern Belle to the roots and a heat protectant like Hot Toddy all over, and comb through to evenly distribute.

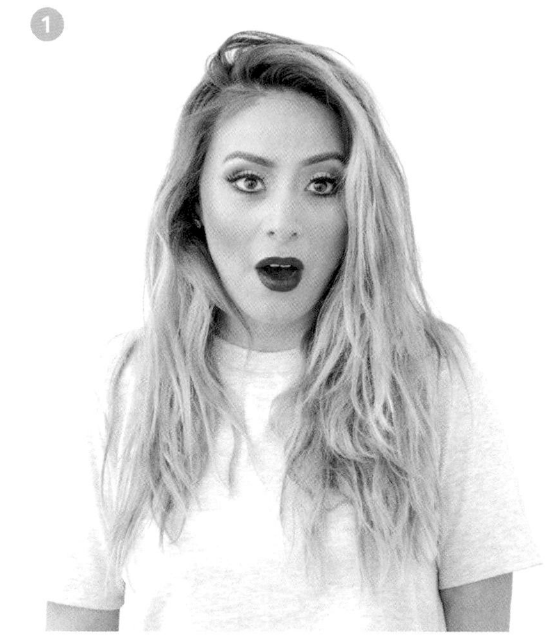

For **soft, fine hair** with a slight natural wave, break out a sea-salt spray like Mai Tai Spritzer and apply at the roots to add grit and texture!

2. After rough-drying, section your hair like a pro. Part your hair as you normally do. Brush the hair that frames your face forward, then draw a clean line from the back of one ear to the back of the other and secure these sections with one clip on each side. Wrap the back into a bun and clip out of the way to keep moisture intact.

3. Starting in the front, use a round barrel brush vertically to pick up hair at the roots, and roll hair in and out, drawing the brush down and away from your face. Keeping tension on the brush, unwind and twist hair to release it when the section is completely dry.

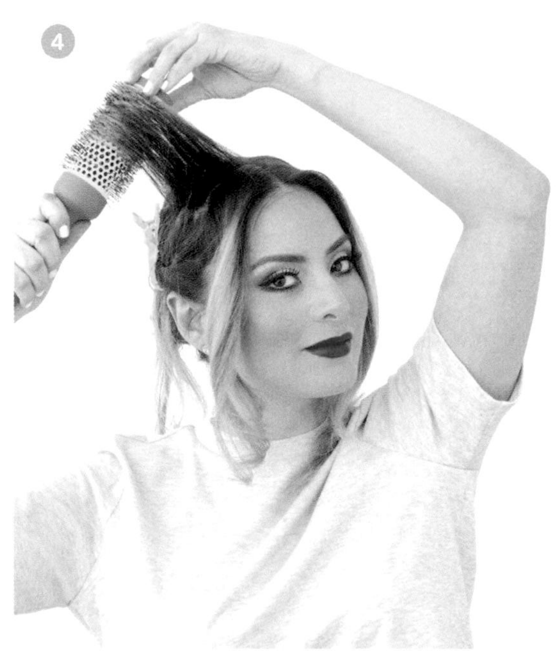

4. Repeat same technique on the next sections and on both sides - working your way towards the crown.

5. To get started on the back, draw a horizontal line from ear to ear, separating the back into two (or three) sections. Always be sure to keep dry hair away from wet hair.

6. Secure the top/crown portion with a clip.

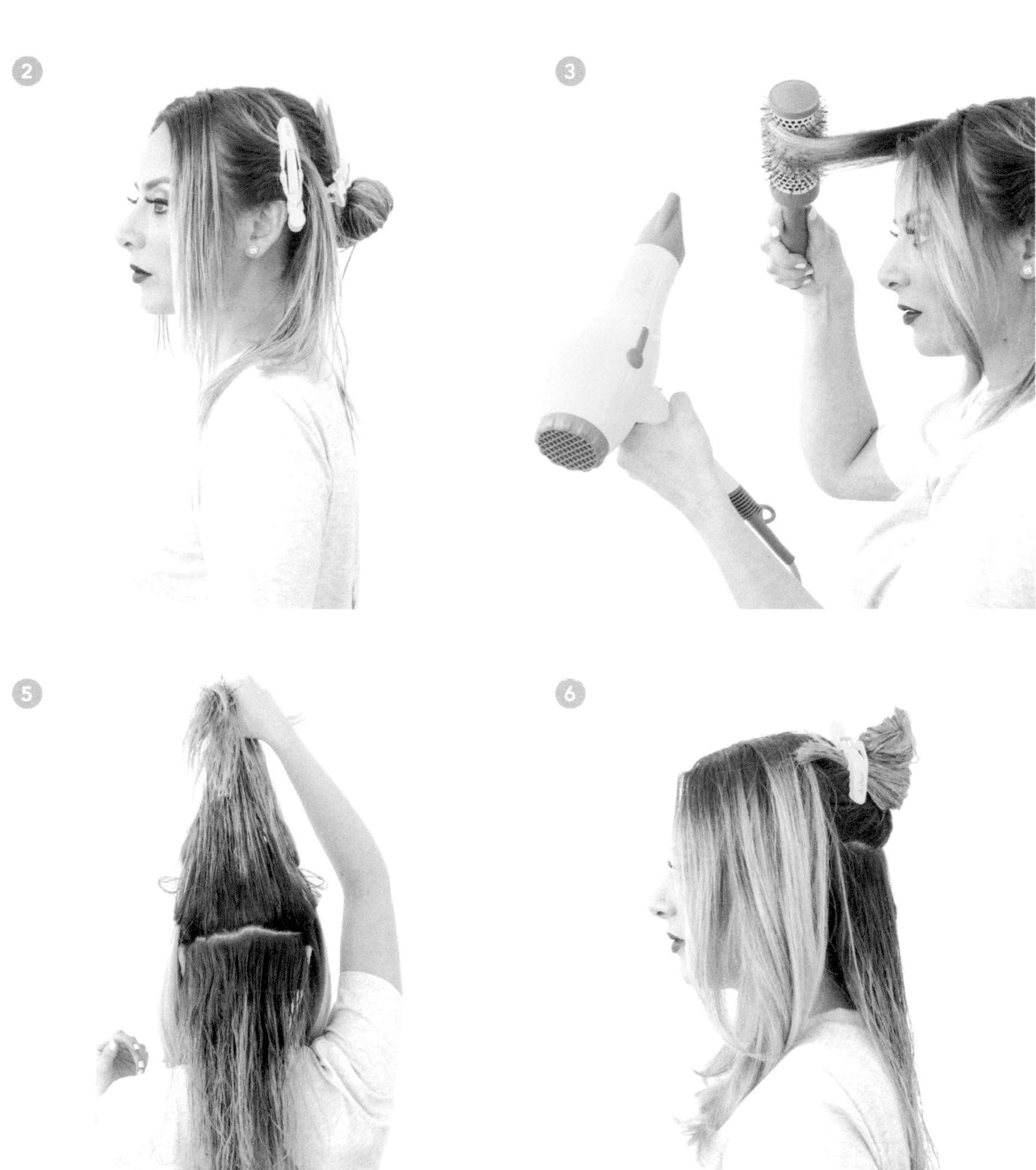
2
3
5
6

7. Working in 2-inch (5-cm) vertical sections using a vertical brush, direct hair from the nape of the neck forward (this works on most lengths), start at the roots and roll the hair in and out vertically, keeping tension on the brush, and twist out to release.

8. The twist is all in the wrist. Think about twirling a sparkler. And don't touch the curls! Allow them to cool and set.

9. Don't worry if your curls aren't perfect at this point. Adding even the smallest amount of wave while you dry will help your hair hold much longer—a trick we always use at Drybar to make blowouts last!

10. To add a bit of volume at the crown, take a large horizontal section of hair, start with the brush firmly at the roots, and roll the hair up and down, from roots to ends, repeatedly to lock and set volume at the crown.

11. Want more, more, more? Use a preheated curling iron to define your curls. Working in manageable 1- to 2-inch (2.5- to 5-cm) sections from front to back, clamp your ends and twist the barrel away from your face, or wrap 2-inch (5-cm) sections of hair around the barrel of a preheated curling iron, hold for just a few seconds, then release.

The longer you let your perfect curls set and cool, the better they will hold up. Use this time to do your makeup instead!

7

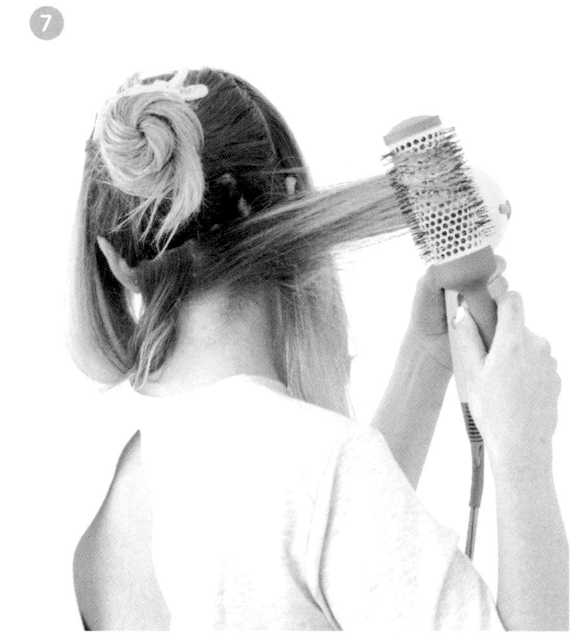

10

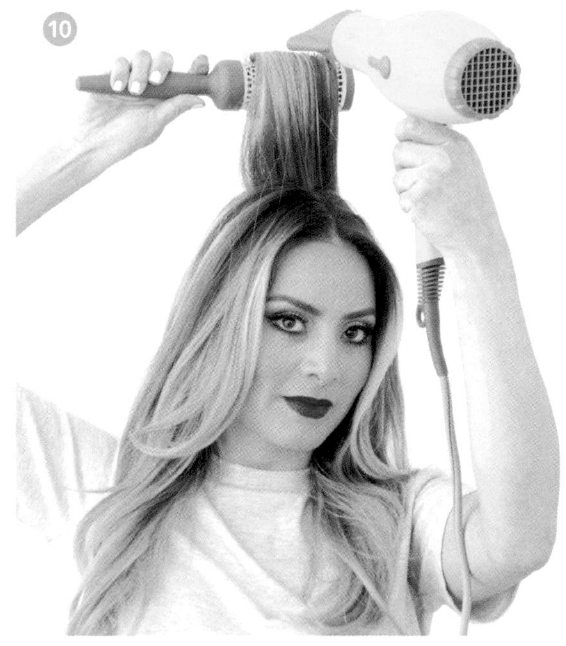

8

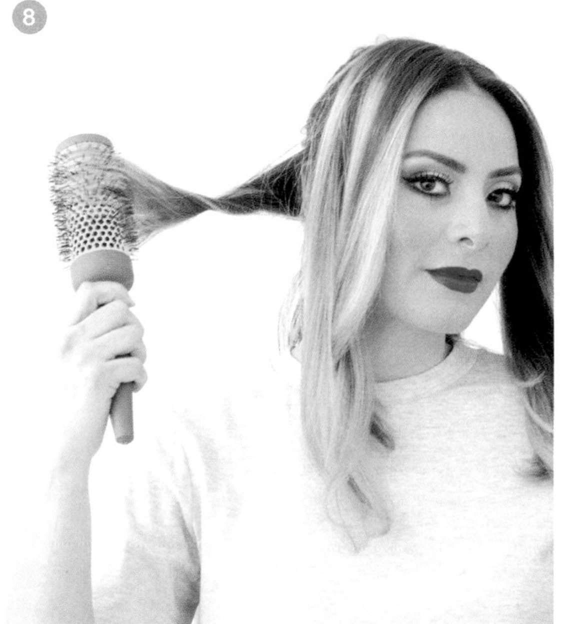

9

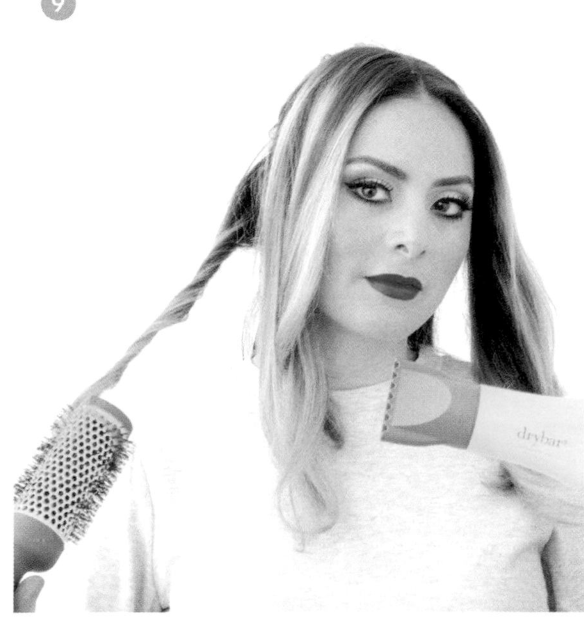

11

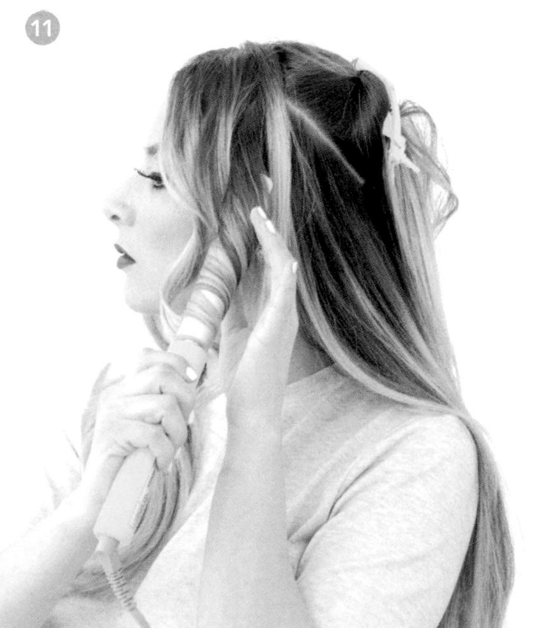

You just can't go wrong with a Cosmo. These big bouncy curls will certainly put a pep in your step as I witnessed time and time again at Drybar.

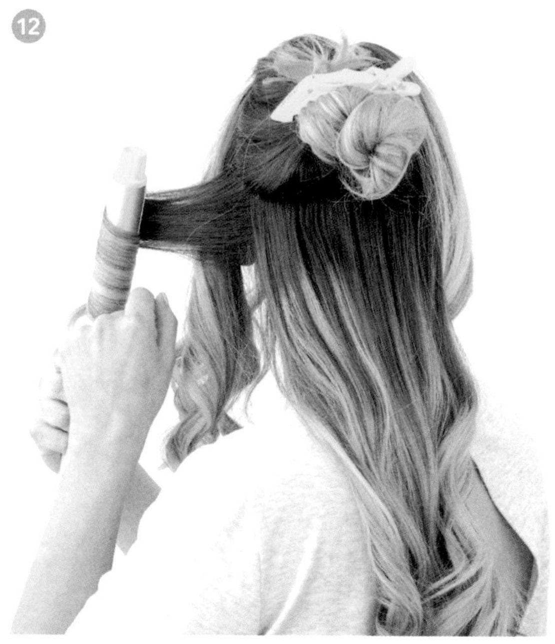

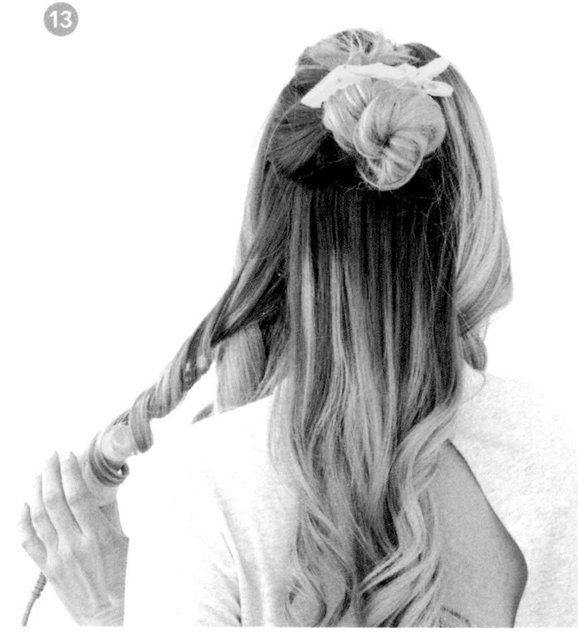

12. If the barrel of your curling iron doesn't rotate, wrap 2-inch (5-cm) sections of hair around the barrel.

13. To maximize the curl, twist to release. Continue curling in vertical sections all the way around your head.

14. For more shine and texture, apply a small amount of shine cream like the Chaser to your ends, and set your style with a firm-hold hair spray like the Sheriff.

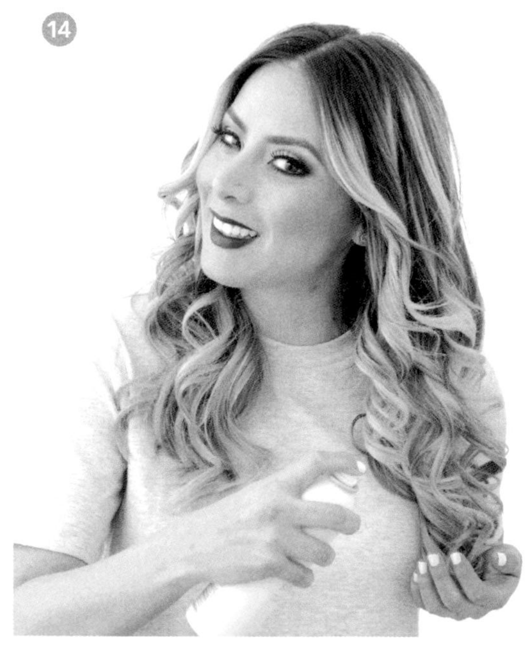

. TIPS .

CURL, YOU KNOW IT'S TRUE

· GET A LITTLE LOOPY ·

For extra oomph, flip your hair, spray with a texturizer like Triple Sec, tousle, and go!

· GIVE IT A WHIRL ·

The way to build lasting curls is to really work it: Always start at the roots. Always use a comfortable amount of tension. Always roll the brush in and roll the brush out. Repetition is the key to a great, long-lasting blowout!

· RINGLET MY BELLE ·

If your curl is too Shirley Temple, loosen the sections by tugging on them while your curls are still warm to soften them up. If that doesn't work, treat the curling iron as a flat iron, clamping down on a section and running the iron through quickly to help straighten things out.

· HAVE YOU SEEN MY CURL? ·

Maybe it's online! Check out our 3-Day Bender video tutorials online for more how-to advice.

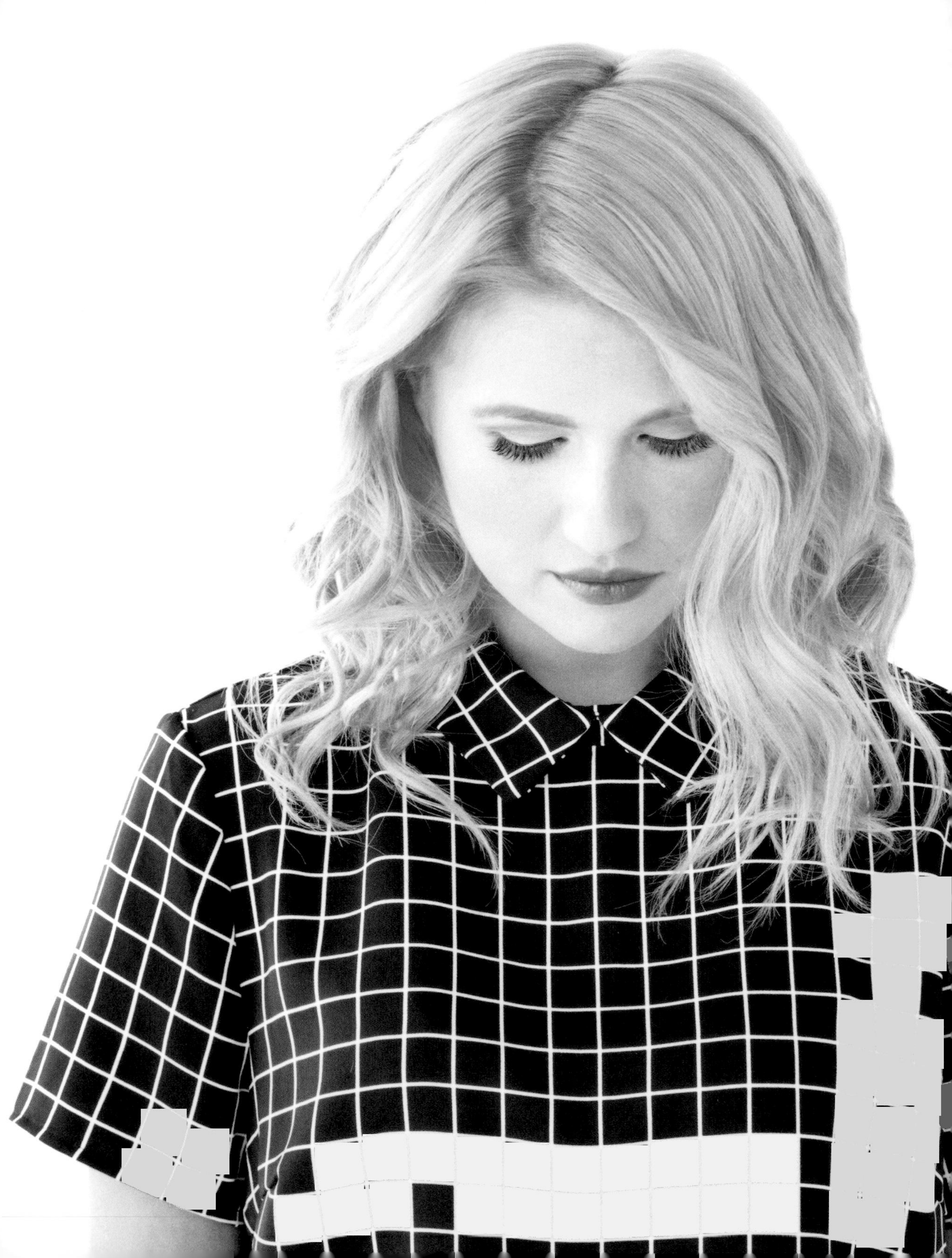

– THE –

MAI TAI

MESSY, BEACHY HAIR

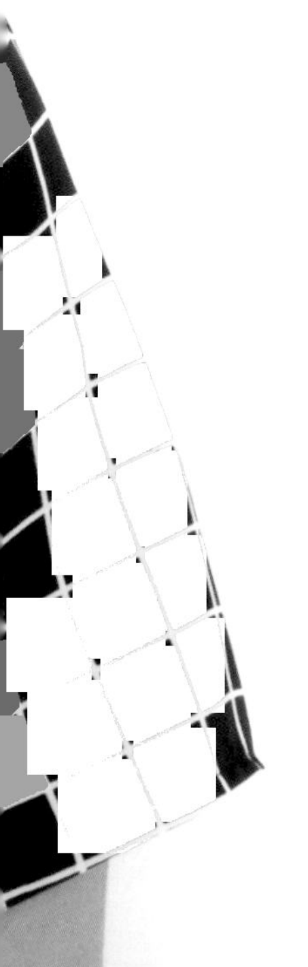

THE
MAI TAI

FOOTLOOSE AND FANCY-FREE

Ingredients:

Leave-in conditioner

Heat protectant

Sea-salt spray

Detangling brush

Blow-dryer

Clips

Small or medium round ceramic-barrel brush

Shine cream

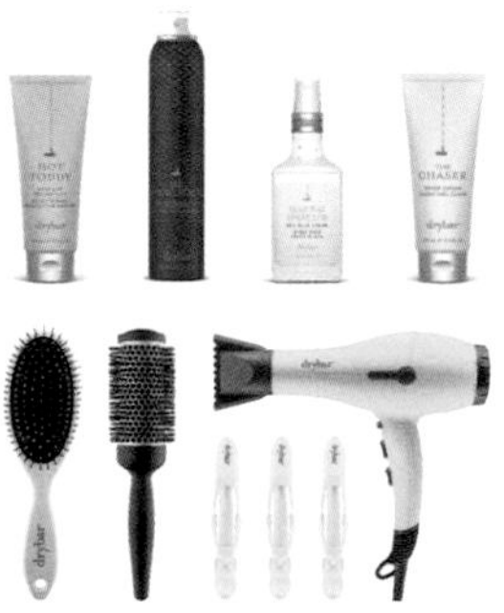

You deserve just-back-from-vacation hair even—no, especially—if you've just spent all day at school, work, with the kids, or just TCB-ing like the super boss you are.

The Mai Tai is one hairstyle that plays especially well with hair that already has a lot of natural texture going on (i.e., mine). With enough product, time, and willpower, you can force your hair to do just about anything, but the Mai Tai is more about working with what you've got.

A free-spirited style like this does not want to be weighed down. For fine hair, pump up the volume with a sea-salt spray or texturizer at the roots. Medium and curly hair won't need much, but if your hair is on the dry side, try a leave-in conditioner before styling to keep frizz at bay. Either way, finish off the look by scrunching shine cream at the roots and ends for fun.

The Mai Tai is perfectly imperfect. Just like us.

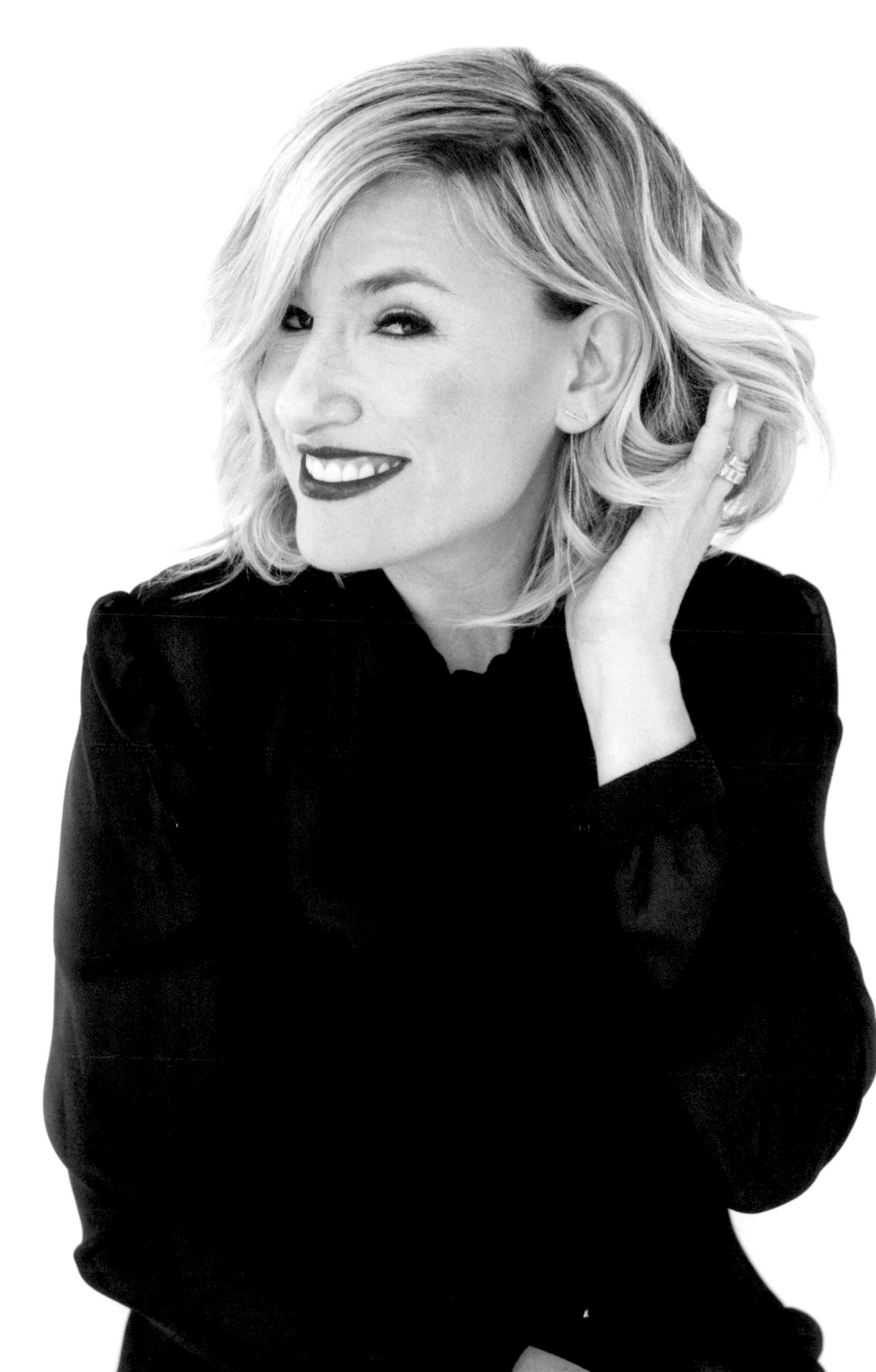

1. Presenting the frizzball (that's me!) that started it all: lots of natural texture, a combo of waves and curls that like to knot, and a tendency toward dryness. Hair jackpot! Not.

2. After towel-drying, apply a heat protectant like Hot Toddy all over or a leave-in conditioner like Mr. Incredible from midshaft to ends and comb product through.

If your hair is **naturally straight**, try a body and texture building product like Texas Tea volumizing spray and a little Mai Tai Spritzer at the roots to give it the grit it needs to hold some curl.

3. With the dryer on high, rough-dry your hair pointing the dryer down the hair shaft, using your fingers to diffuse the airflow and create movement. For extra texture and body, try tossing the hair around a bit.

4. Draw in your part and section out the front of your hair—ear to ear and forward. Clip the rest out of the way.

5. Using a small or medium round barrel brush (smaller brush, more curl; medium brush, less curl), blow bangs dry by picking up a horizontal section from your part and rolling the brush from roots to end forward and away from your face. Release the ends with a twist of the wrist and let the curl cool and set.

1

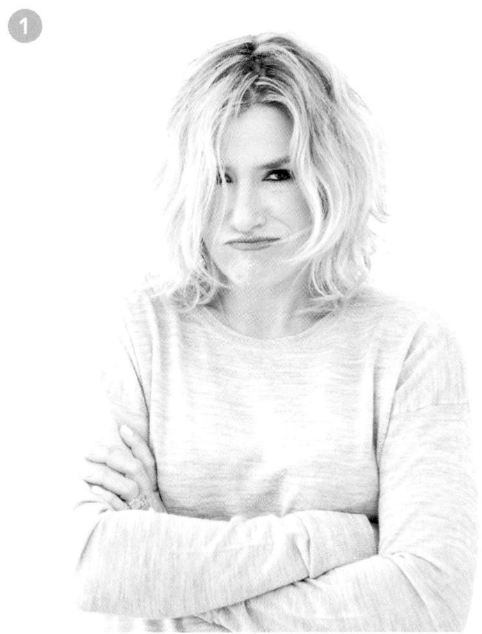

4

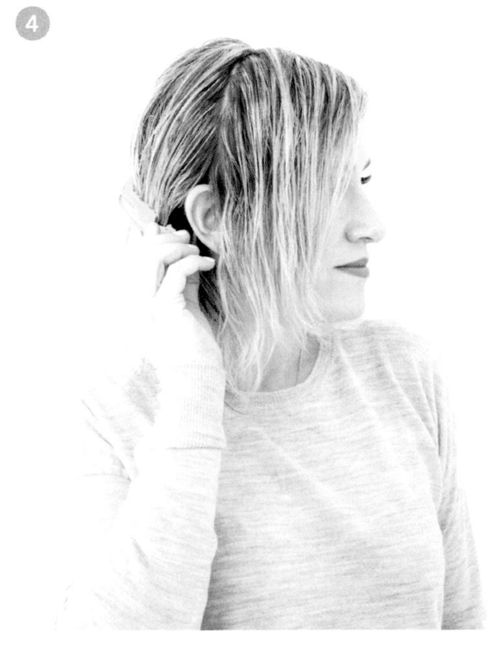

2

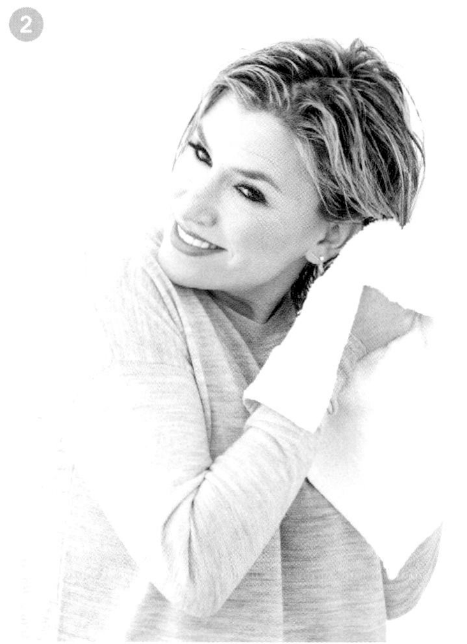

3

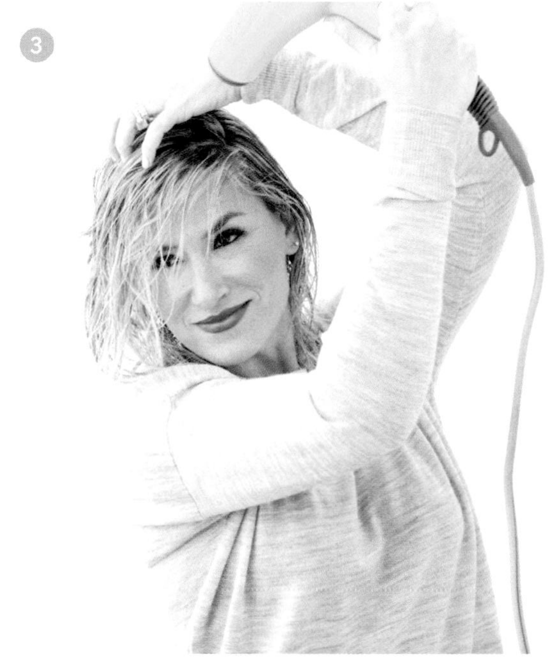

5

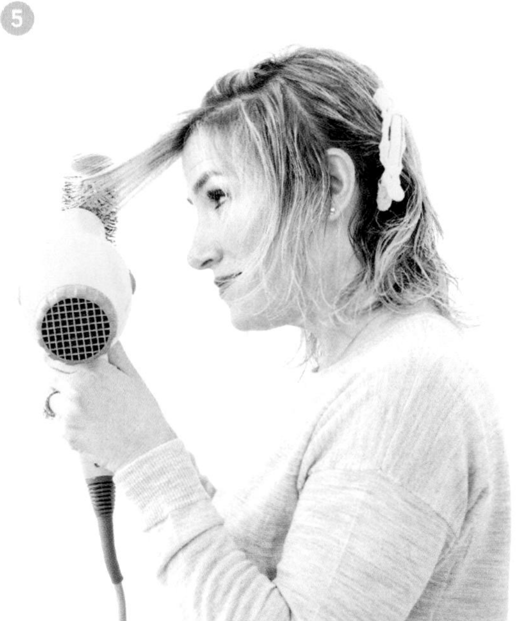

Keep your friends close and your hair clips closer. Boy, do those things come in handy!

6. To frame your face, pick up vertical sections at the roots and roll through to the ends, moving away from your face, and twist to release. I prefer to hold the handle down, but if it's more comfortable for you to hold the handle up, go for it! Just be sure to twist out the brush so your curl stays intact.

7. Working in vertical subsections from your part, pick up hair at the roots and roll to the ends, angling the brush up and back to create wave and volume.

8. The more twist you give the brush, the longer lasting the curl you build in will be. That's the name of the game, ladies!

9. Divide the back of your hair into two sections. Clip the top section up and away. Working in vertical sections, continue to pick hair up at the roots and roll from roots to ends, twisting to release.

10. If your hair is on the shorter side and vertical sections won't stay on the brush, no sweat, just work subsections at an angle to create some movement.

11. Now, using your round ceramic-barrel brush, pick up larger sections of hair and roll the brush vertically from roots to ends, maintaining tension the whole time.

What's Quackin'? I always slip a duck-bill clip into my bangs to help set my part without getting indentations.

6

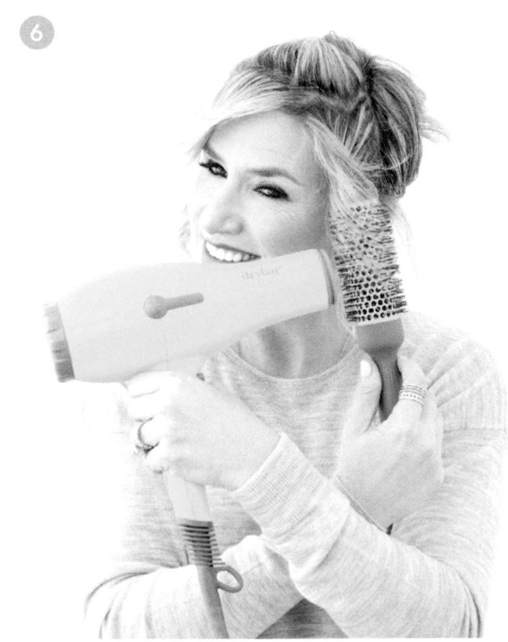

9

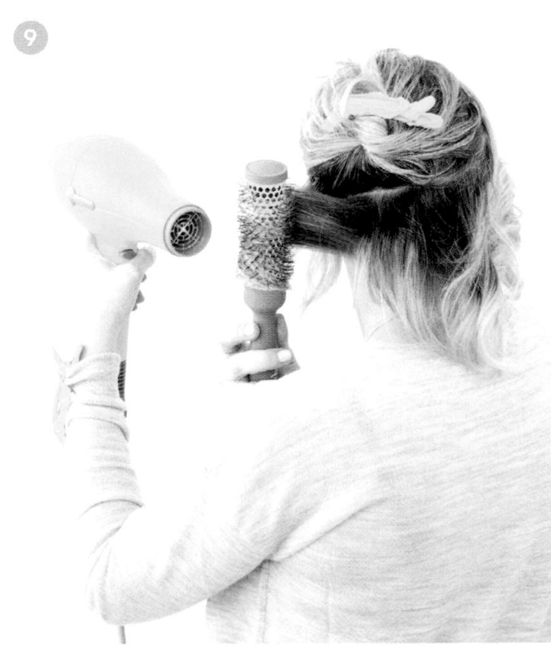

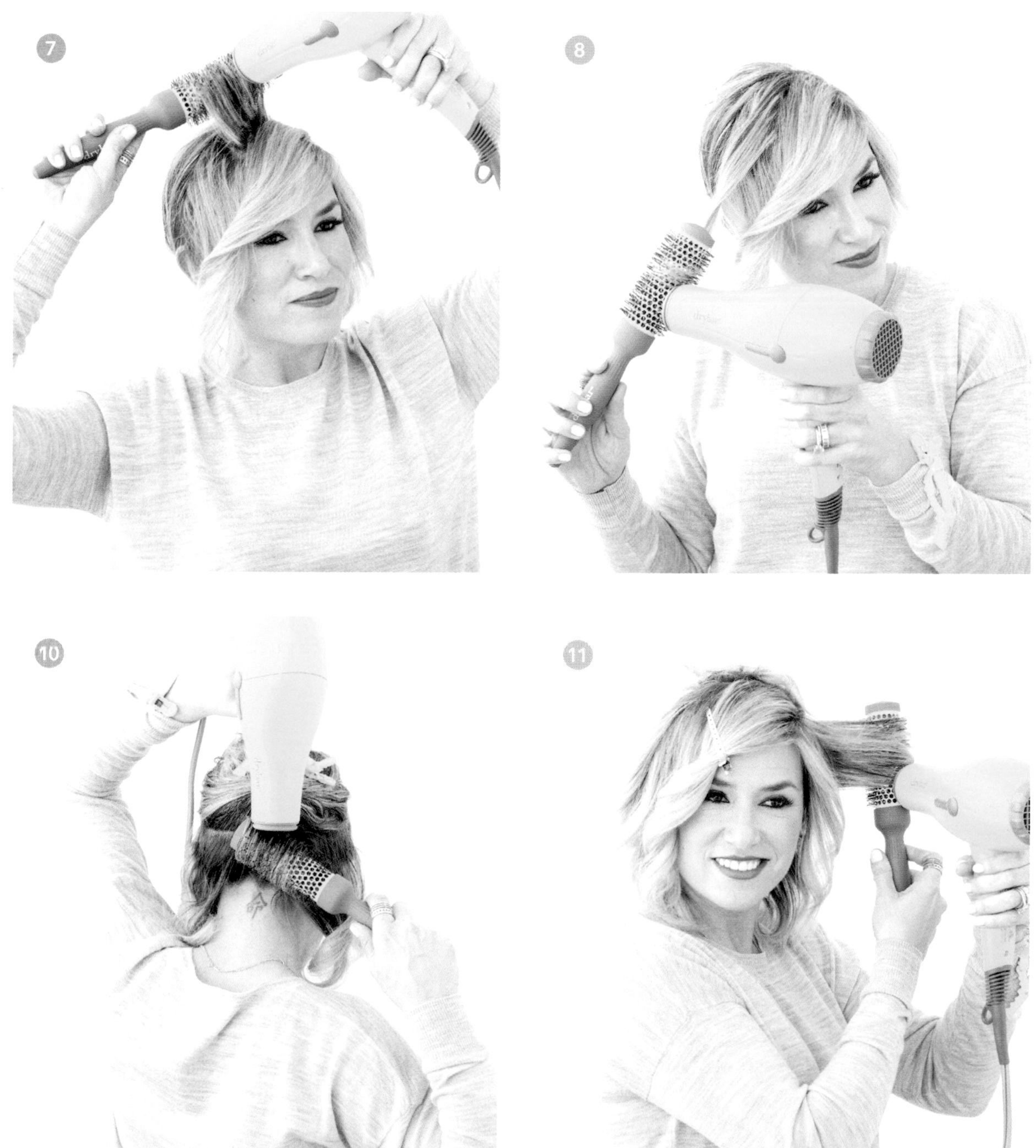
7
8
10
11

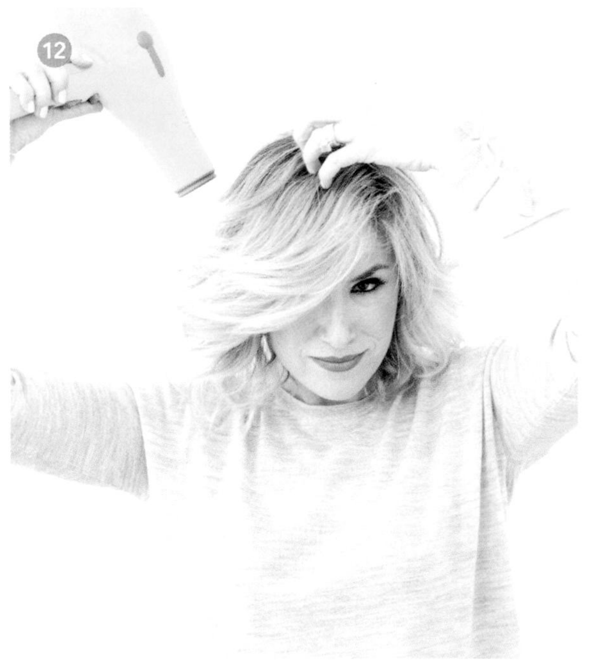

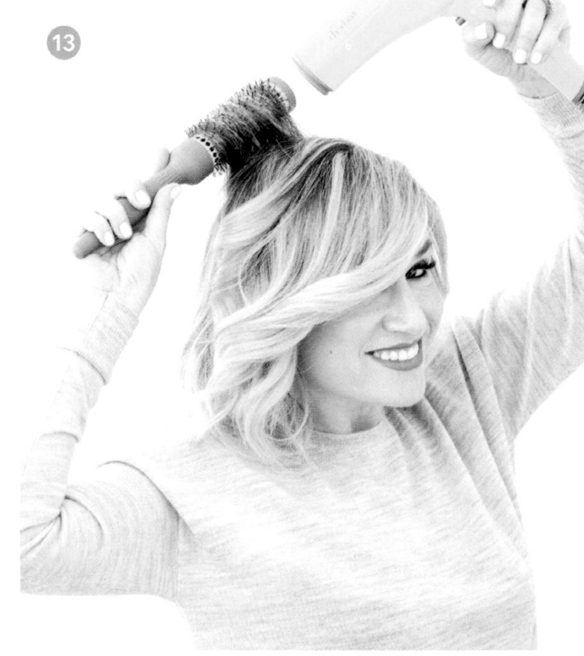

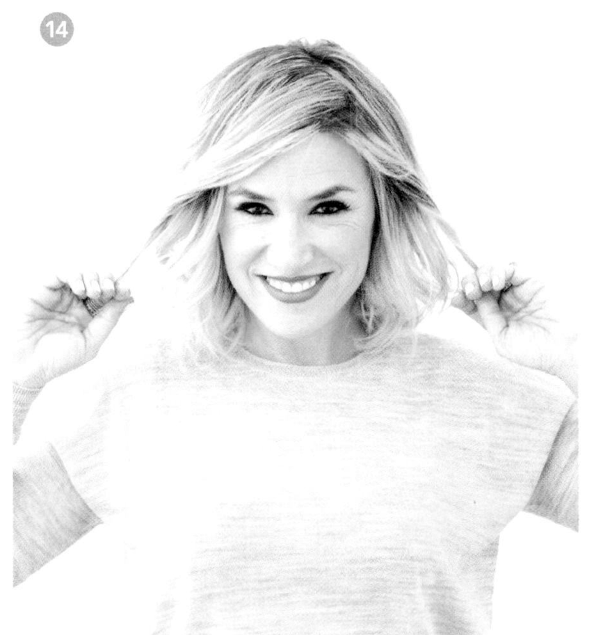

12. Once you've built in all the curl, blow it apart to loosen it up and see where things land.

13. To add volume at the crown, pick up horizontal sections at the roots and roll the brush from roots to ends, angling the brush up and out. For even more volume, set the hair with a Velcro roller.

14. To finish the look, add a small amount of a shine cream like the Chaser to the palm of your hand, rub hands together, and twist small sections of hair around the face for a tousled, piecey look.

· TIPS ·

IT'S NOT JUST MAI TAI, IT'S EVERYBODY'S TAI

· STRAIGHT TALK ·

Some hair just doesn't want to hold a curl. For straight hair that seems to want to stay that way, build in the curl with a round brush as you blow-dry. Finish with a texturizing spray like Triple Sec or Mai Tai Spritzer.

· A CLUE FOR HUES ·

Color-treated hair takes less time to dry! When rough-drying, aim to remove only about 30–40 percent of the moisture so that you can still manipulate the hair and set the style how you would like.

· SUN KISSED ·

You know you nailed the Mai Tai when you look like you just walked off the beach, only better (and less sandy). Perfect for when you want to feel laid-back, yet look super chic.

· UNDER ONE CONDITION ·

Coloring, processing, or using the wrong products can all damage and dry out your hair. Adding a hydrating hair mask to your routine once a week will help nurse your mane back to health.

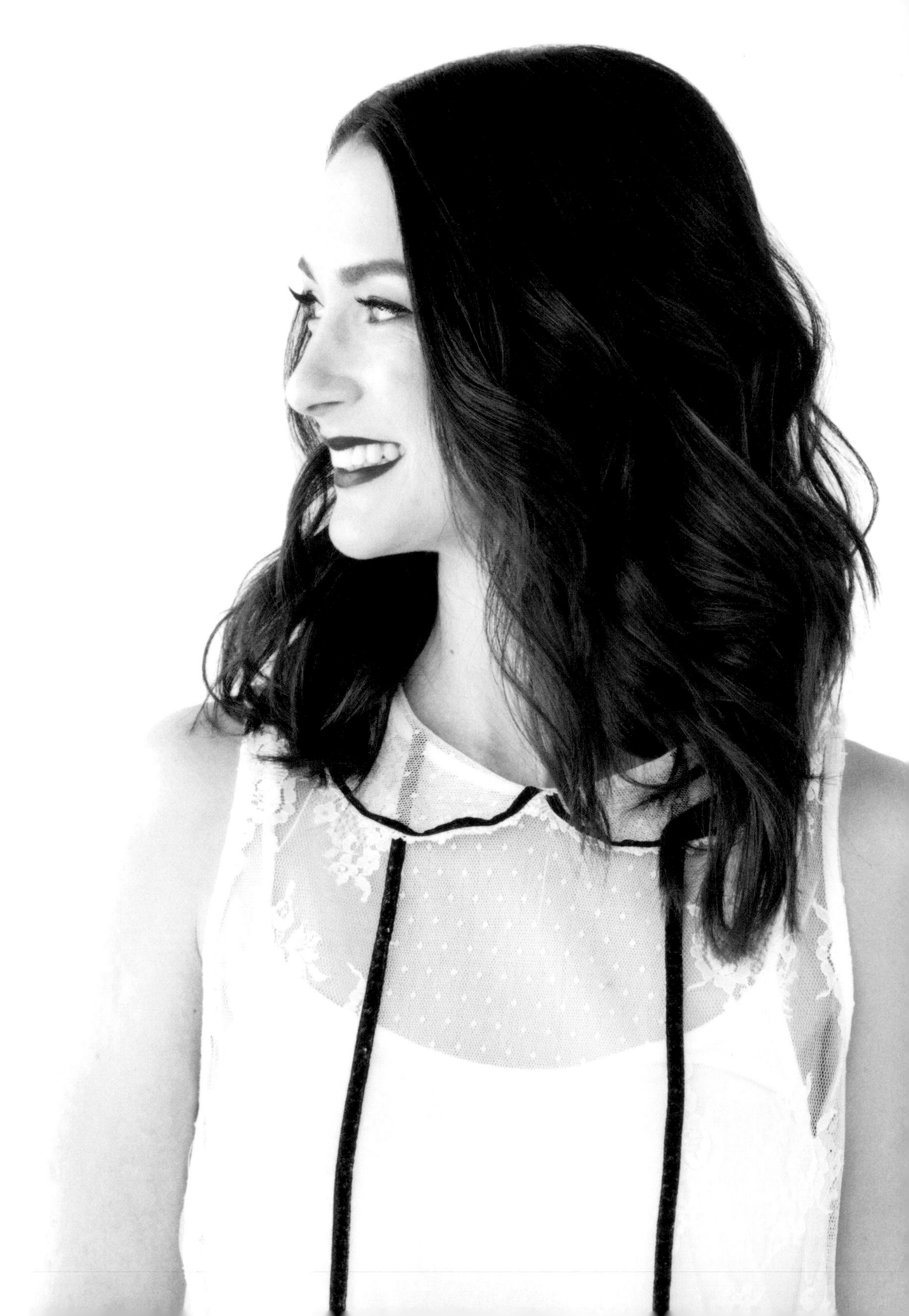

- THE -

COSMO-TAI

A LITTLE COSMO, A LITTLE MAI TAI

THE COSMO-TAI

IT'S THE BEST OF BOTH WORLDS

Ingredients:

Heat protectant

Hydrating control cream (for my curly/coarse/frizzy ladies)

Sea-salt spritzer

Detangling brush

Blow-dryer

Clips

Small round ceramic-barrel brush

Medium or large round ceramic-barrel brush

Large self-grip roller

Curling iron

Shine cream

Firm-hold hair spray

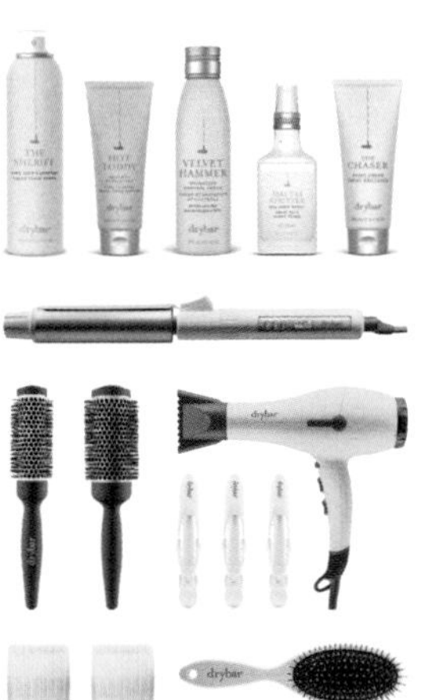

What do you get when you cross a Cosmo with a Mai Tai? No, not a hangover (but good guess). The answer is hair that's full of body and movement, with curls that are just shy of defined.

Not as sculpted as a Cosmo and not as freewheeling as a Mai Tai, a great Cosmo-Tai can be nailed more easily than you think. If your hair is fine and straight, concentrate on creating nice lift at the roots and good body and curl all around, so you'll still have style going even if your curl starts to fall out. If your hair has natural wave, use as little product as you can get away with and work on getting the hair nice and smooth, so that when you break up your curls they relax nice and easy.

With the Cosmo-Tai, you can have it all.

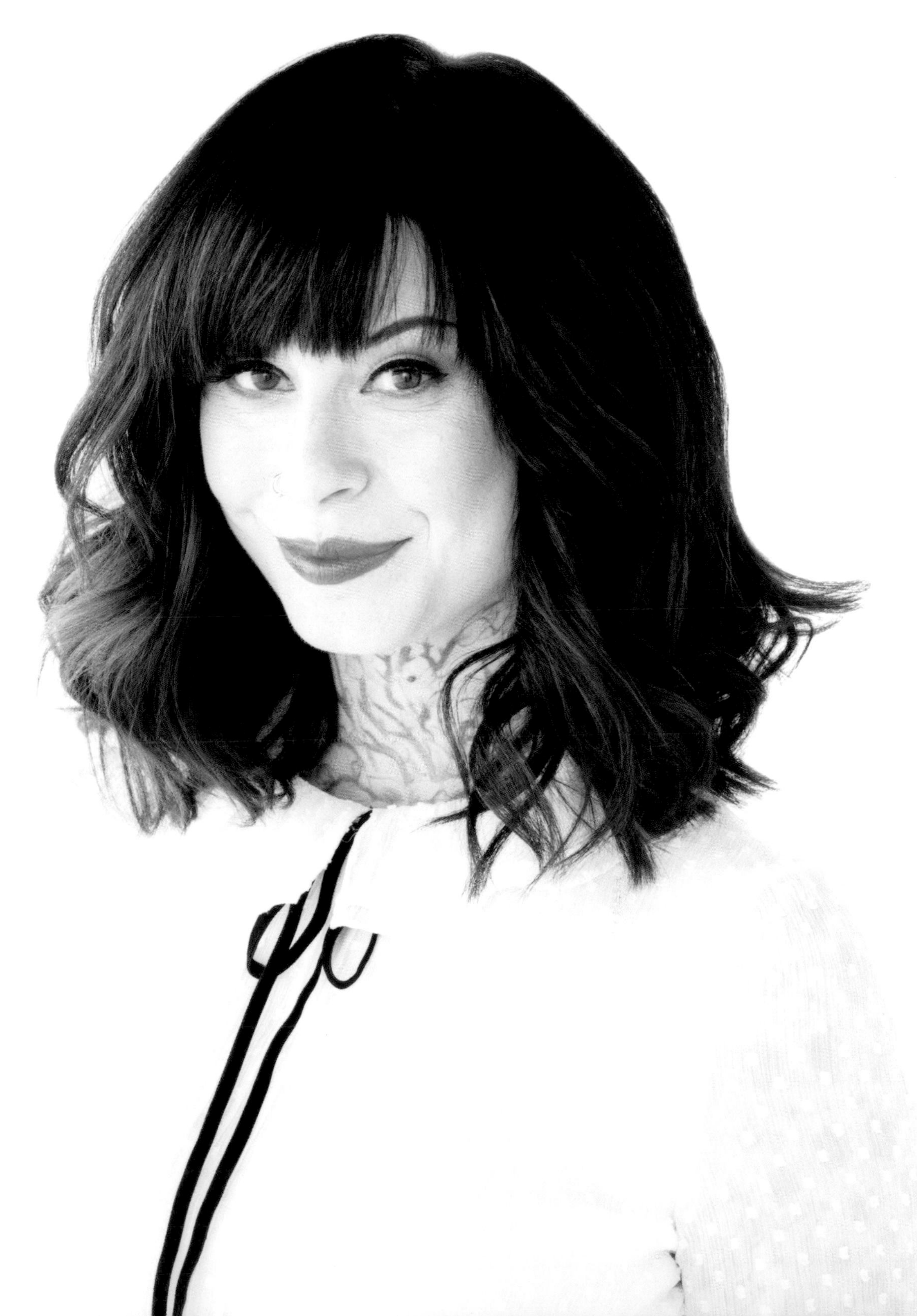

1. Thick hair can be a blessing (the way it is in fairy tales, when you're a princess and you need to grow your hair super long so your prince charming can climb up it and rescue you) and a curse (say, when you are late for work and your hair is soaking wet and will stay wet until lunch unless you blow-dry it).

2. After towel-drying hair, apply a heat protectant like Hot Toddy from roots to ends and follow with a hydrating control cream like Velvet Hammer, applied from midshaft to ends; then brush through to distribute evenly.. Part your hair and rough-dry bangs, using your fingers to help direct the fringe and neutralize any cowlicks.

If you have **fine hair**, you want a product that will help build volume and hold. Try a volumizing mousse like Southern Belle or a texturizing spray like Mai Tai Spritzer so your Cosmo-Tai stays put.

---

3. When bangs are involved, section out the bangs and clip wet hair back away from your face.

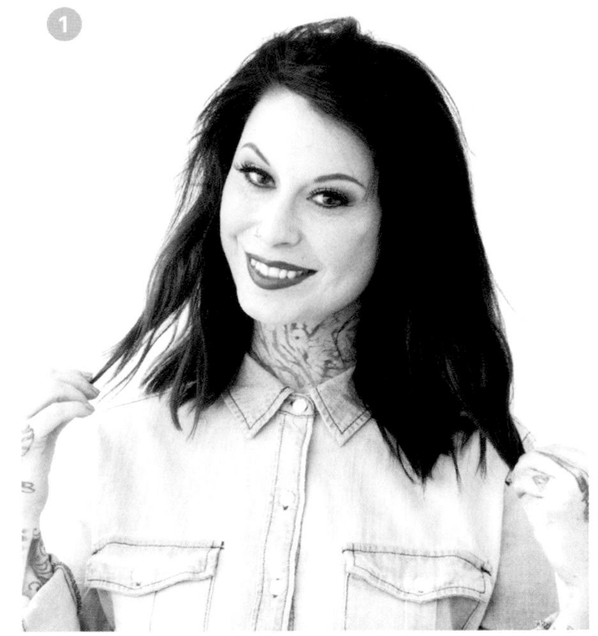

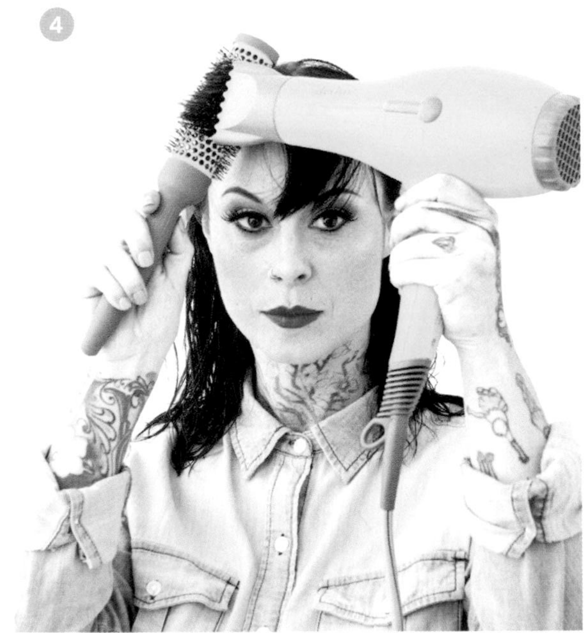

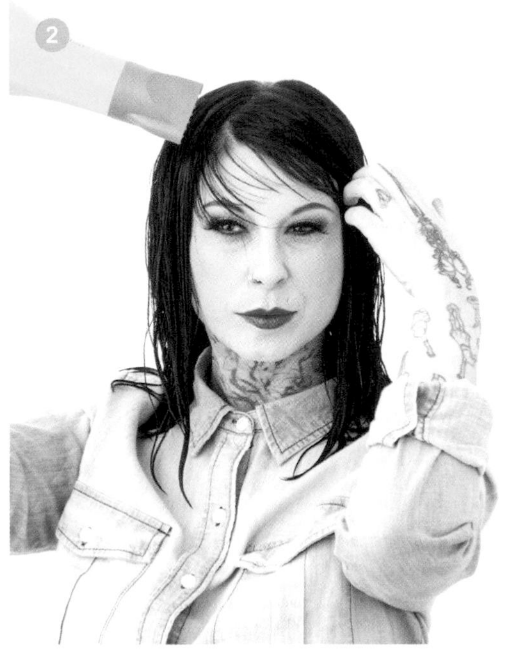

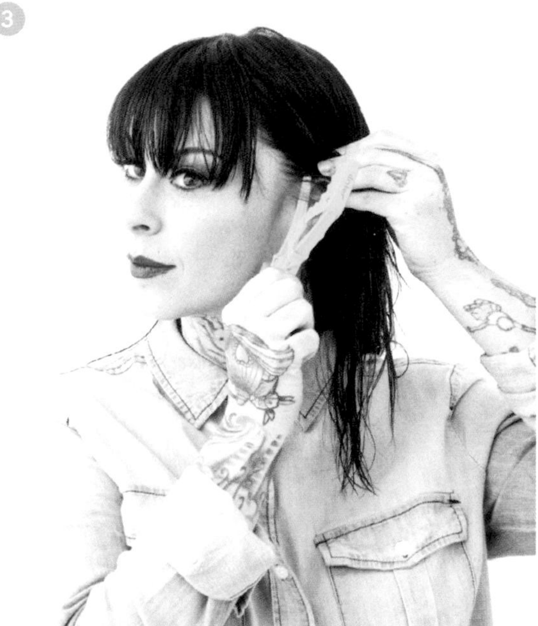

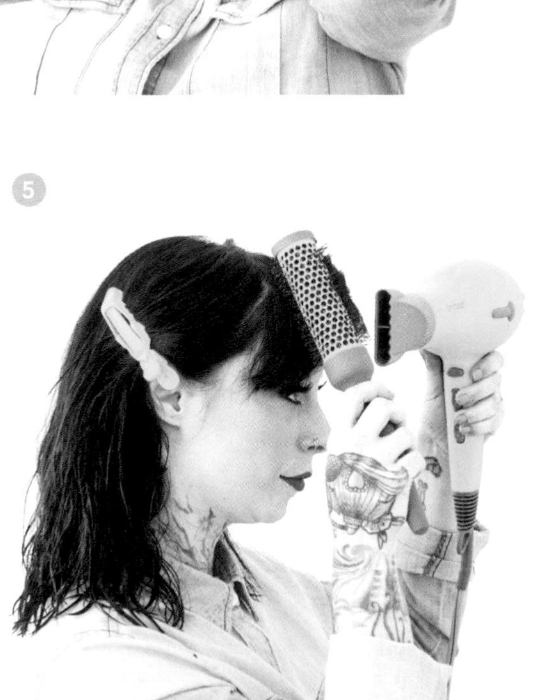

4. Using a small round ceramic-barrel brush, work in small subsections to blow bangs dry in vertical sections.

5. Keep slight tension on the brush to blow bangs away from your face. Avoid placing the brush horizontally underneath bangs or you'll wind up with a poofy bangs bump.

6. Once bangs are dry, section out the front of your hair, from ear to ear forward, and clip the rest back.

7. Now switch to a medium ceramic-barrel brush for longer hair. Holding the brush vertically, pick up 2-inch (5-cm) sections of hair from behind and roll the brush from roots to ends, angling it back and down, creating a slight wave.

Tool Time: If you have **shorter** hair, or just **more curl**, stick with a small ceramic-barrel brush!

8. To build lift, pick up the section of hair at the crown and roll from roots to ends, over directing the hair forward and up. Once this section is dry, wrap ends around a large barrel brush and roll back and down to the roots. Repeat until completely dry.

9. Now let it set. The longer you let your hair set and cool, the longer the volume will last.

10. A large self-grip roller will also do the trick (and is especially handy if you don't have more than one big brush).

11. For even more hold, spray with a firm-hold hair spray.

6

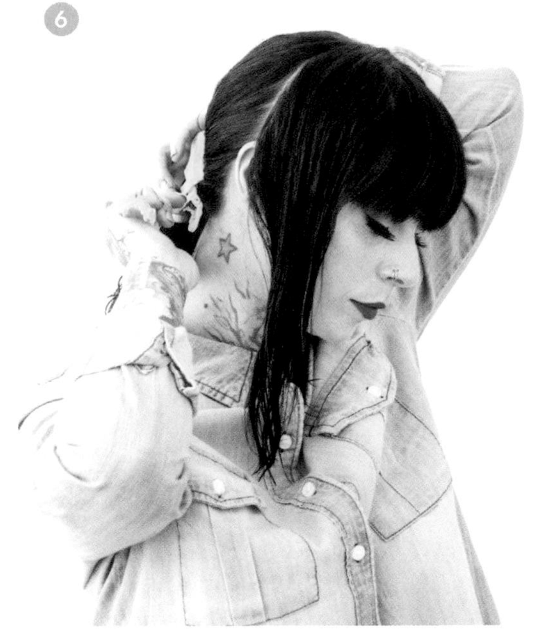

9

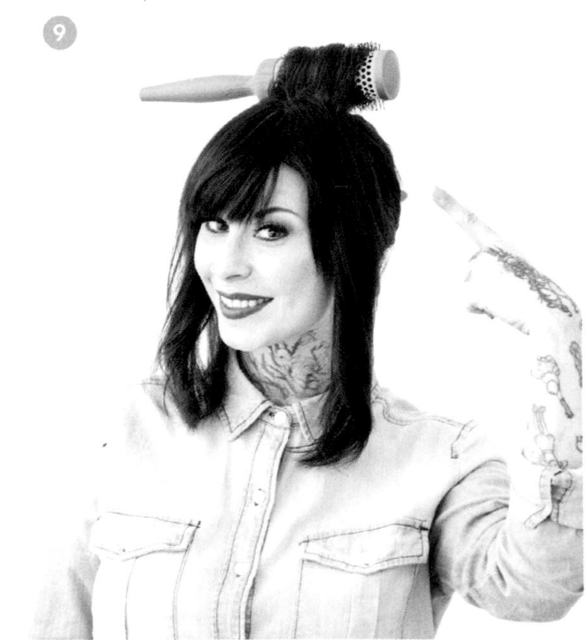

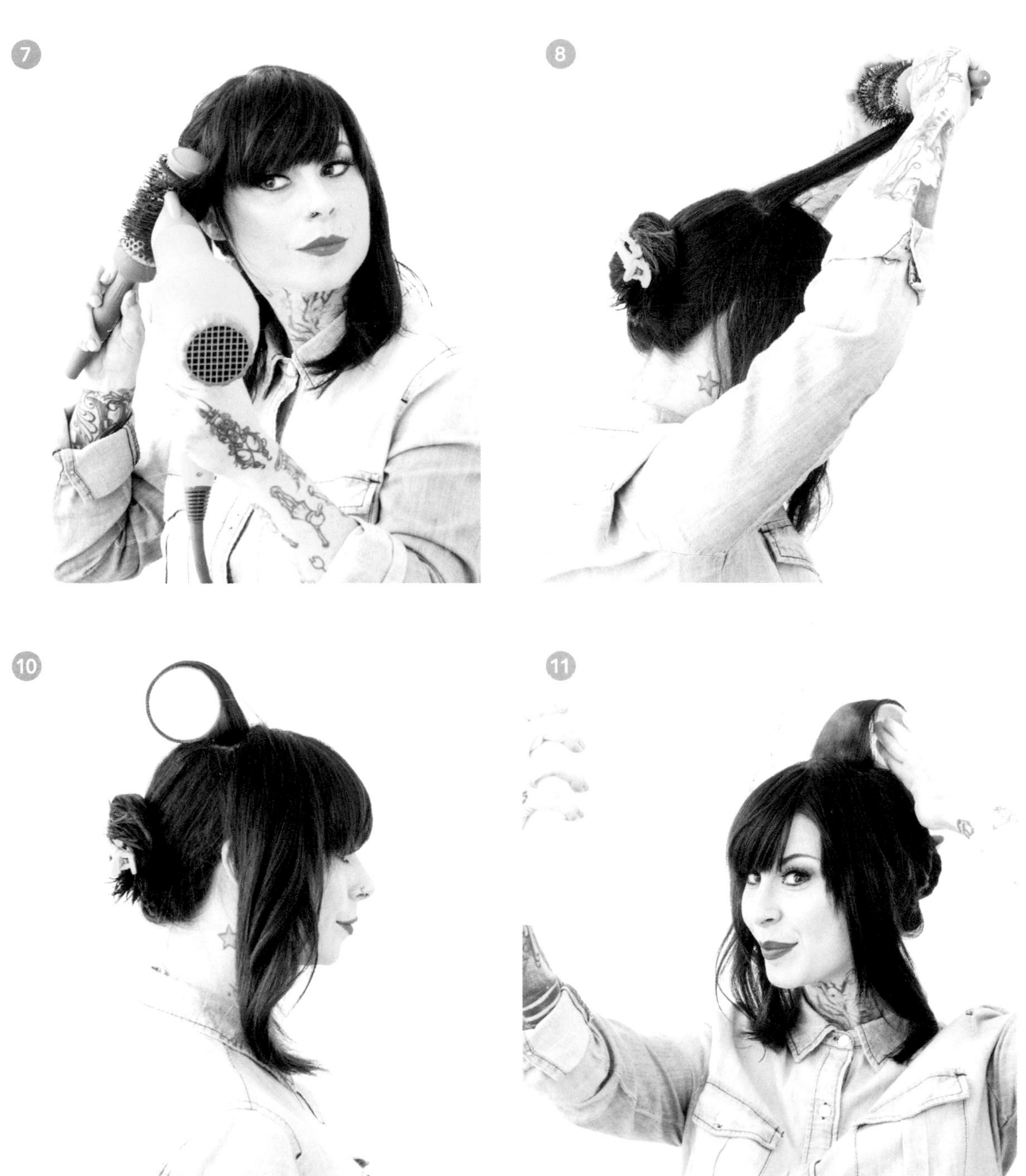
7
8
10
11

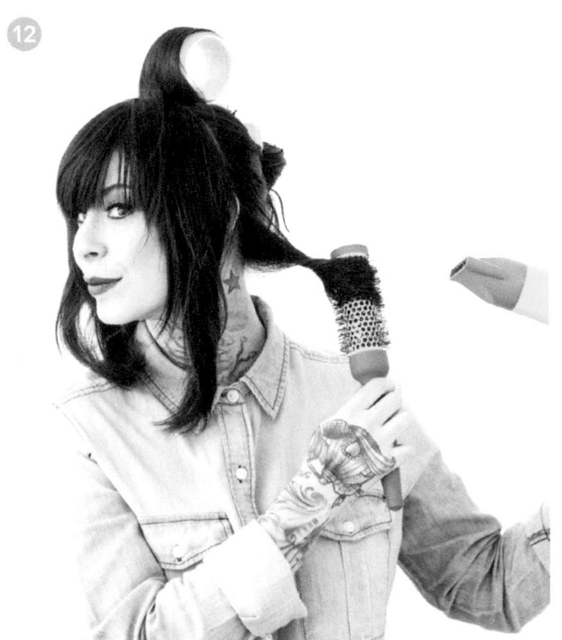

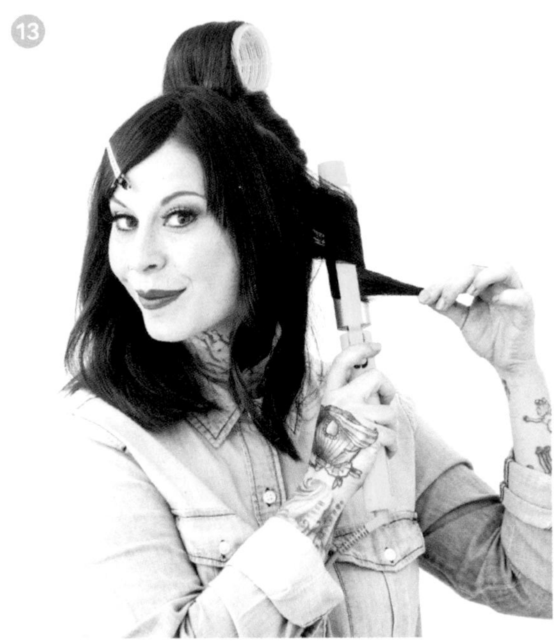

12. Divide the back of your hair into two horizontal sections. Starting with the lower half of your head, pick up vertical subsections at the roots and roll from roots to ends, releasing each section with a twist of the wrist. Repeat on both sides until the back is dry.

13. Add more defined curls with a curling iron like the 3-Day Bender. Taking vertical sections, clamp the iron at the midshaft and wrap around the iron stopping 1 to 2 inches (2.5 to 5 cm) from the ends.

14. To finish it off, take a small amount of shine cream like the Chaser in the palm of your hand, rub hands together, and scrunch through hair to separate curls and loosen things up.

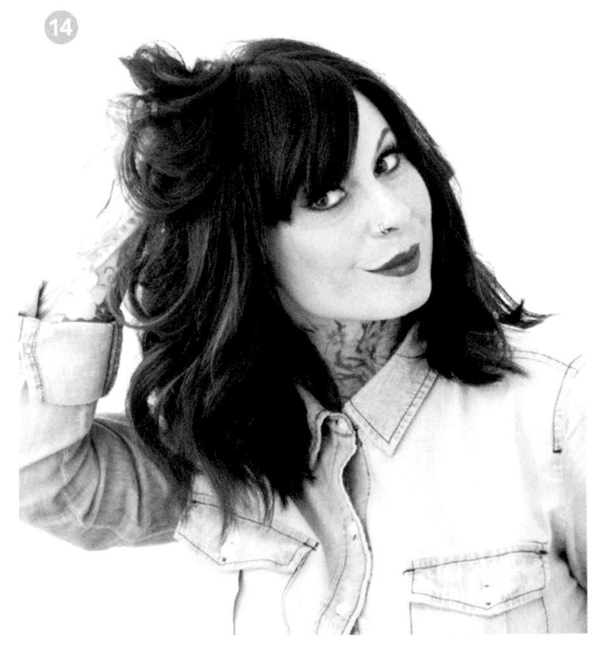

HAIR FLATLINING? CALL FOR HELP!

IF YOUR HAIR FALLS FLAT, TIP YOUR HEAD OVER, SPRAY ALL OVER WITH HAIR SPRAY OR TEXTURIZING SPRAY, AND MASSAGE AT THE ROOTS TO BUILD VOLUME. IT'LL BRING YOUR HAIRSTYLE BACK TO LIFE IN A FLASH.

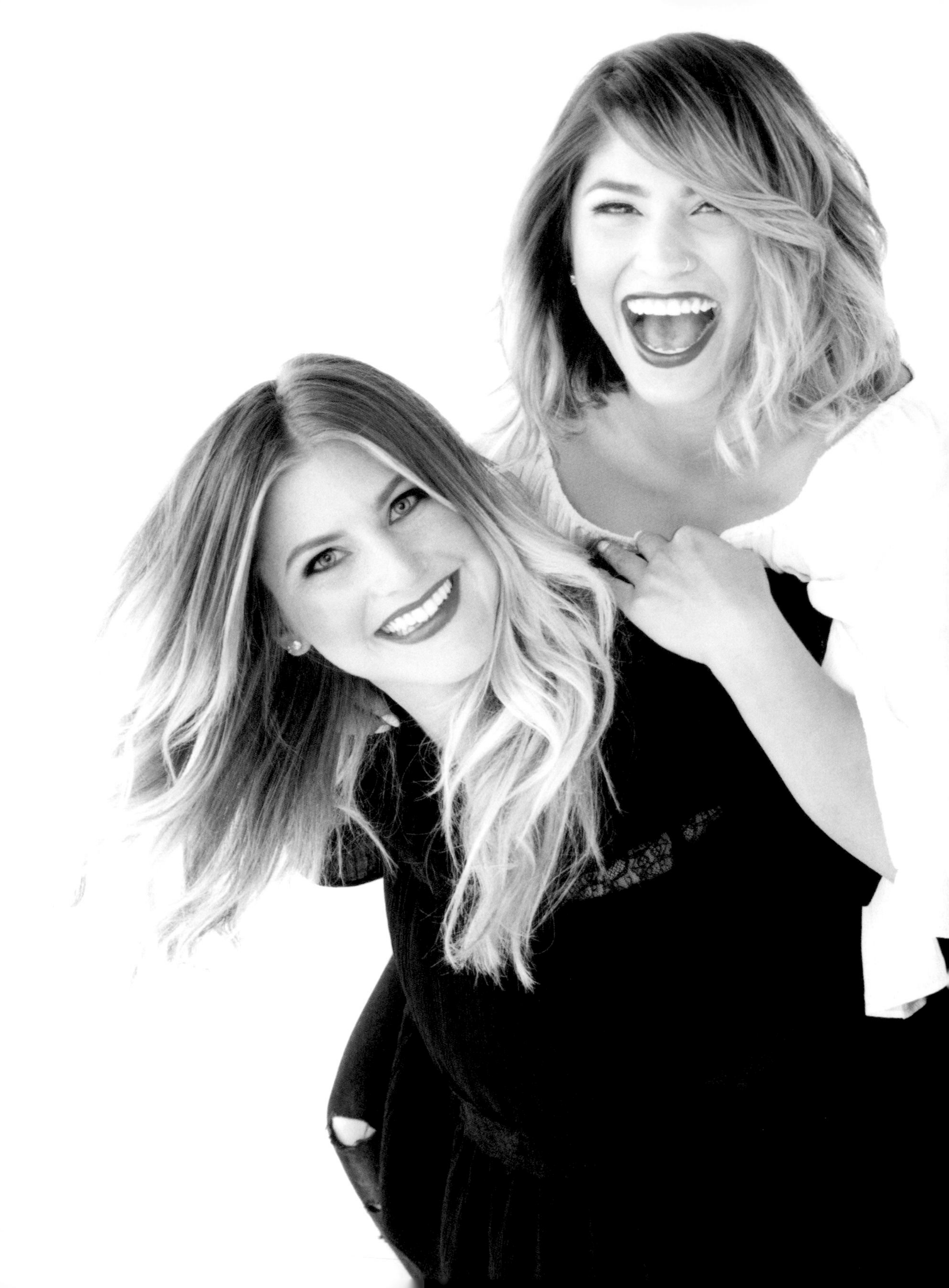

THE DIRTY MARTINI

TOUSLED AND TEXTURED

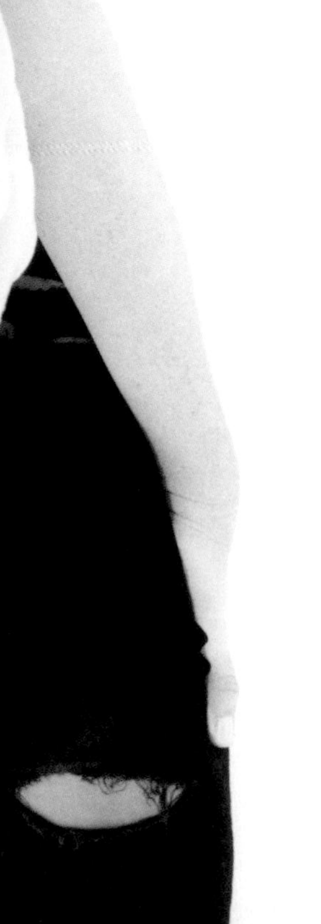

THE DIRTY MARTINI

SOME HAIR RULES ARE MEANT TO BE BROKEN

Ingredients:

Heat protectant

Texturizing spray

Sea-salt spray

Detangling brush

Medium round ceramic-barrel brush

Clips

Blow-dryer

Curling iron

Shine cream

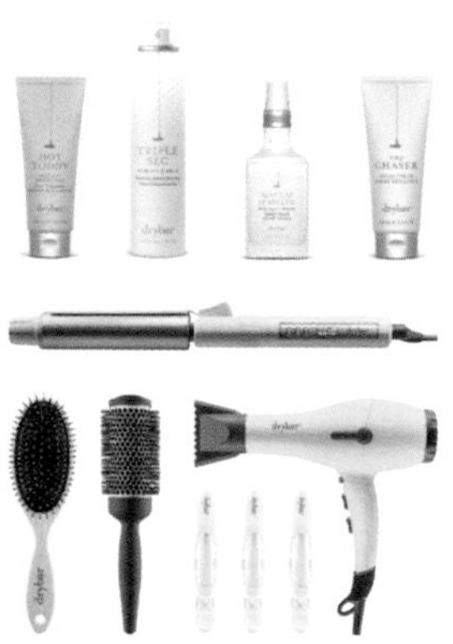

Meet the Dirty Martini: the un-hairstyle. A riskier, more undone look, the Dirty Martini says, "I tried, but not too hard." But under closer examination, you'll see there is no frizz at the roots, there're no fried ends, and there's movement all around. Underneath the too-cool-for-school facade, it's actually all smooth, soft waves and built-in texture.

Depending on your hair type, apply volumizing mousse or texturizing spray at the roots to help build oomph. A shine cream worked in at the roots and ends, or a shine serum only at the ends, will polish it up. When you're finished, it might not look like you've styled your hair at all. And that's when you know you've got it really right.

It's like the best of second-day hair on day one.

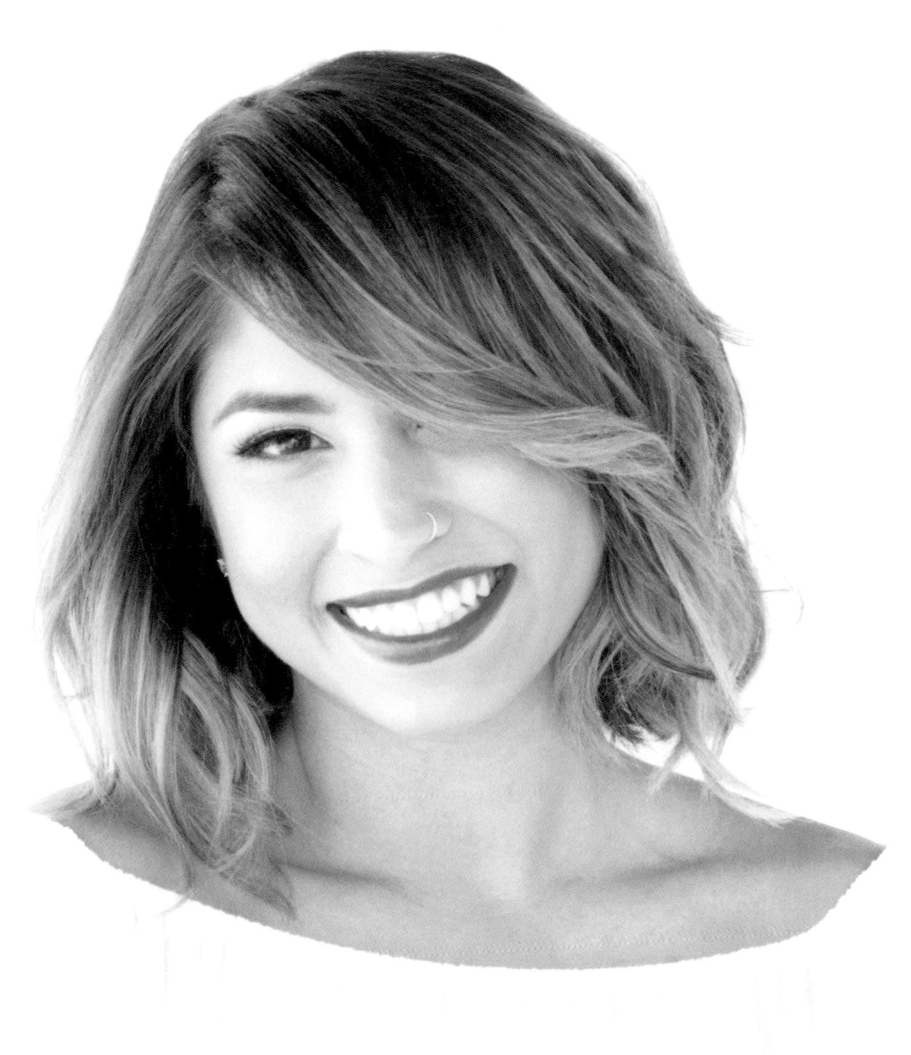

1. Naturally straight hair might seem like a blessing—but not when it has a case of the blahs. A curling iron is key to adding the zhuzh it needs.

2. After applying a heat protectant like Hot Toddy from midshaft to ends, spray a texturizer like Mai Tai Spritzer from midshaft to ends and comb through. This cocktail will give just the right amount of grit and texture needed to build body on straight hair. Sectioning hair will make it easier to dry your hair, but since this style is perfectly imperfect, there's no need to obsess over it.

If your hair has lots of natural **texture** and **wave**, use a volumizing mousse like The Chaser or a hydrating control cream like Velvet Hammer to give roots a boost without going overboard.

3. Start in the front and work your way back. Using a medium round ceramic-barrel brush like the Full Pint, pick up manageable 2-inch (5- cm) sections at the roots, and blow it up and away from the face. Back and forth, again and again—you know the drill.

1

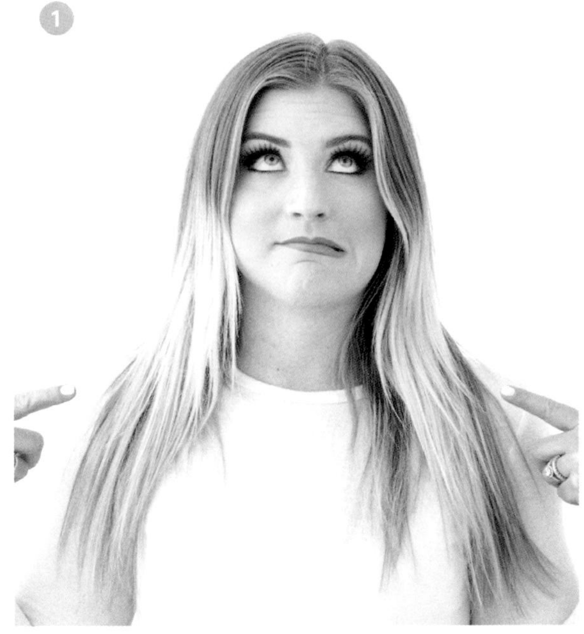

4

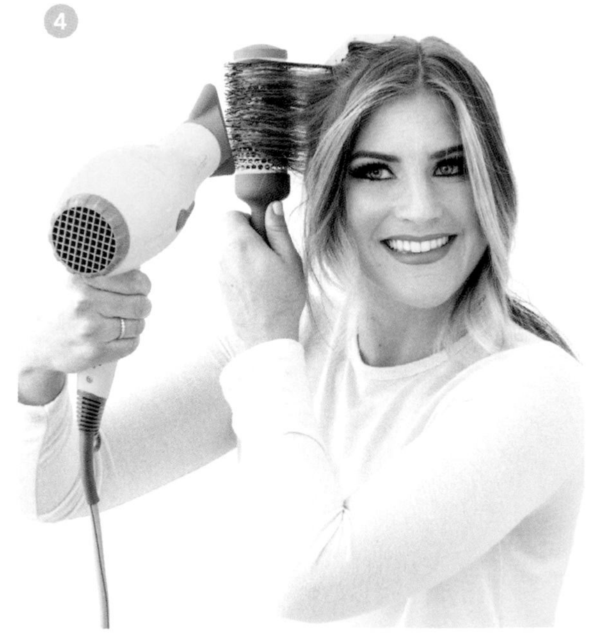

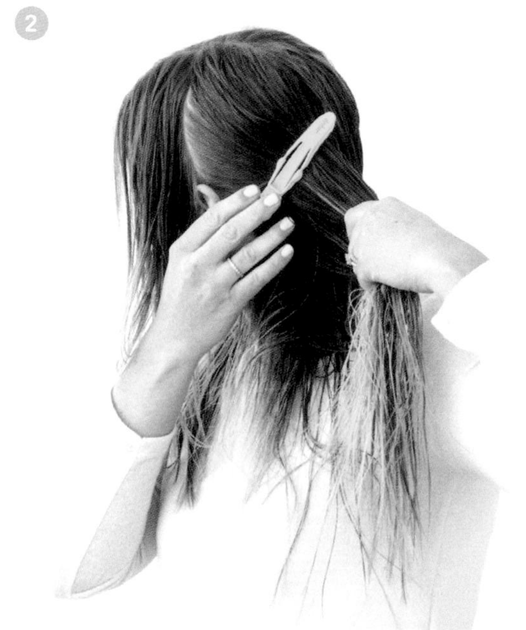

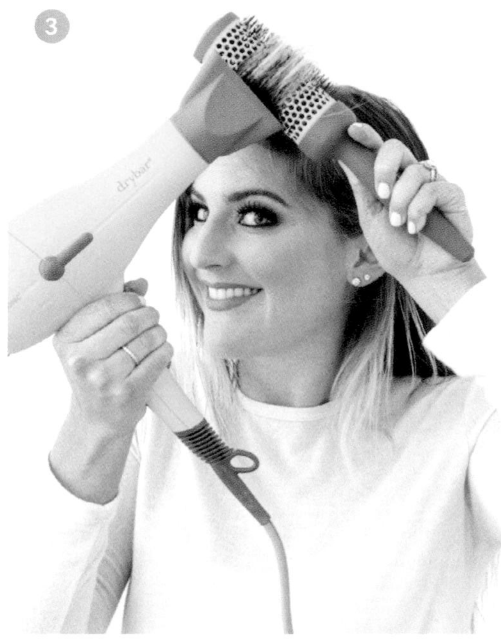

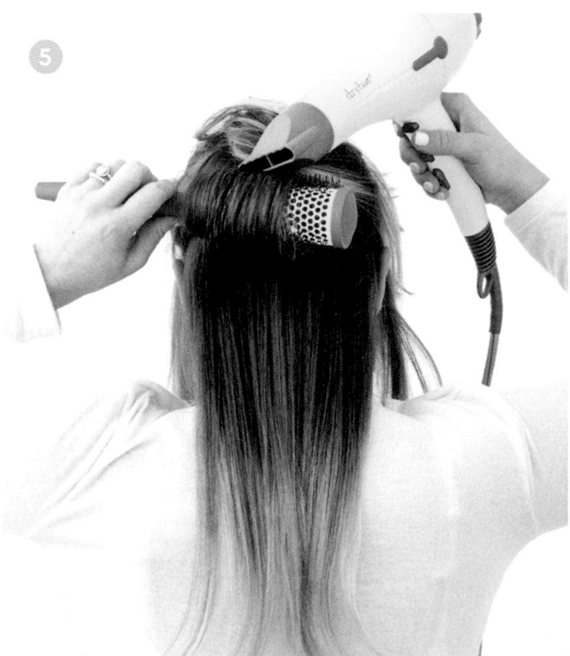

4. Hold the brush vertically as you blow-dry to give the section a bit of bend and body.

5. Once the front is finished, blow-dry horizontal sections of hair from roots to end, creating as much bend/wave/body as you can. I know, I know, it's super challenging for all my straight-haired ladies—don't stress, we have ways around this, I promise.

6. Now that blow-drying is complete, it's curl time. Using a preheated large barrel (use a smaller iron for short hair) curling iron like the 3-Day Bender, curl sections of hair starting at the midshaft. Leave the ends out to score messy points.

7. Work your iron in multiple directions to keep the curl nice, loose, and effortless.

8. Hold the curling iron in at high heat for only a couple of seconds—any longer and the curl could become overly defined.

9. After curling, mist hair with a texturizer like Triple Sec to help bump up the body plus a little hair spray to make curls last. Make sure to spray products up and into the hair, not just on the surface.

10. To turn your curls into loose waves, pull pieces apart and tug on the section once you release the iron.

11. In one hand, combine a small amount of shine cream like the Chaser with a short spray of flexible-hold hair spray like Money Maker, rub palms together, apply to ends and twist.

6

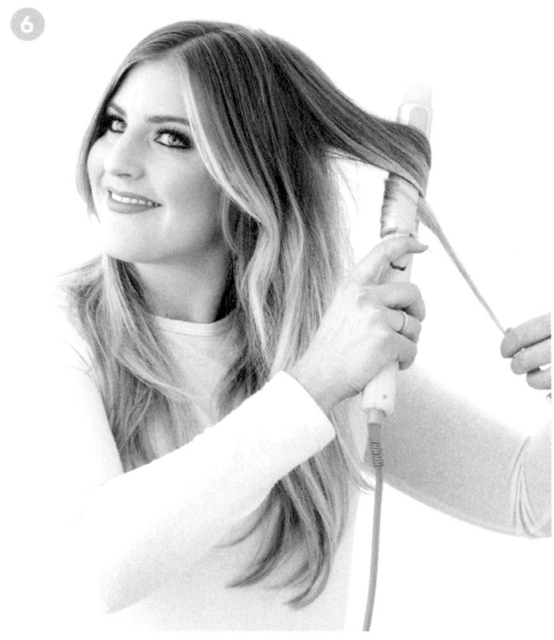

9

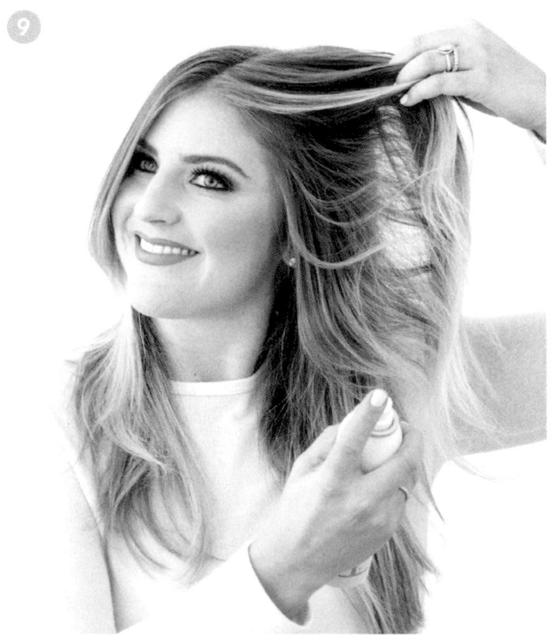

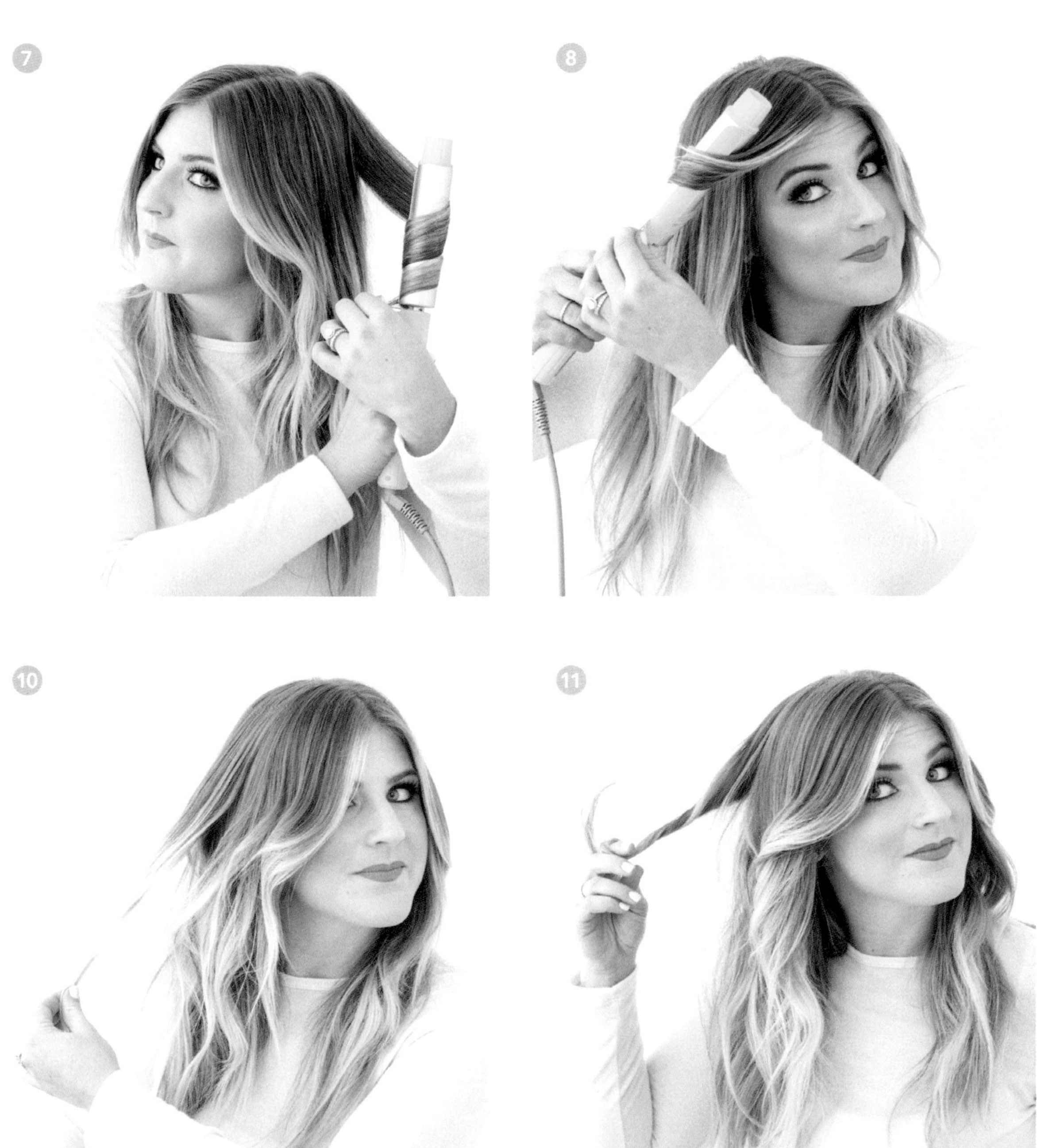
7
8
10
11

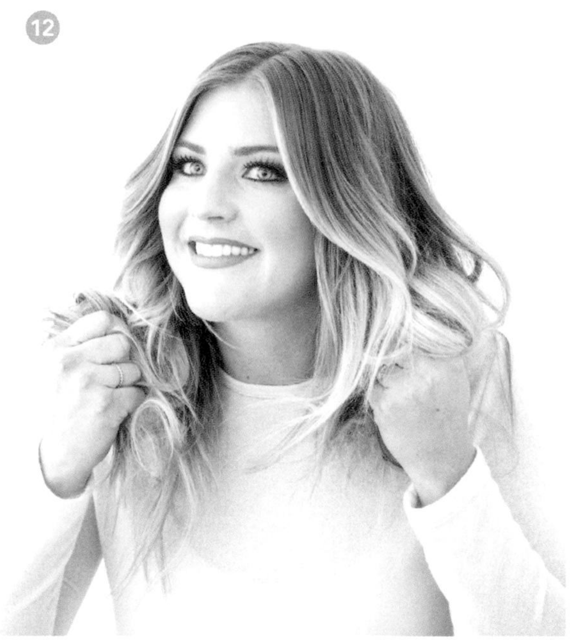

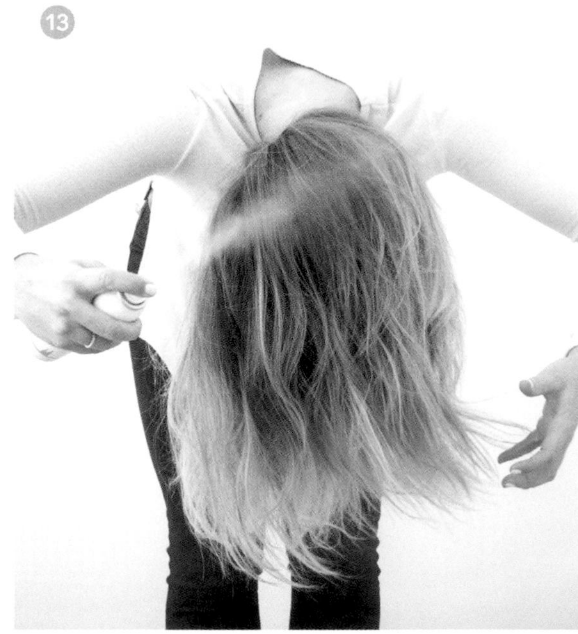

12. Scrunch ends for a more piecey look with movement.

13. Flip hair upside down and spray with a texturizer like Triple Sec.

14. To add volume at the roots, scrunch hands just behind ears and above the nape of the neck. Finish feeling wild and free.

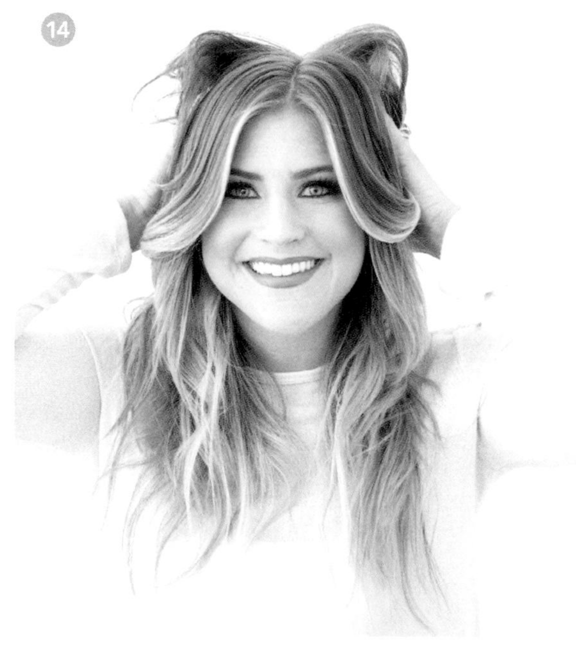

OCD?

WHILE BLOW-DRYING, DON'T SWEAT IT IF YOUR SECTIONING ISN'T PERFECT. **THE DIRTY MARTINI WAS MEANT TO COME UNDONE!**

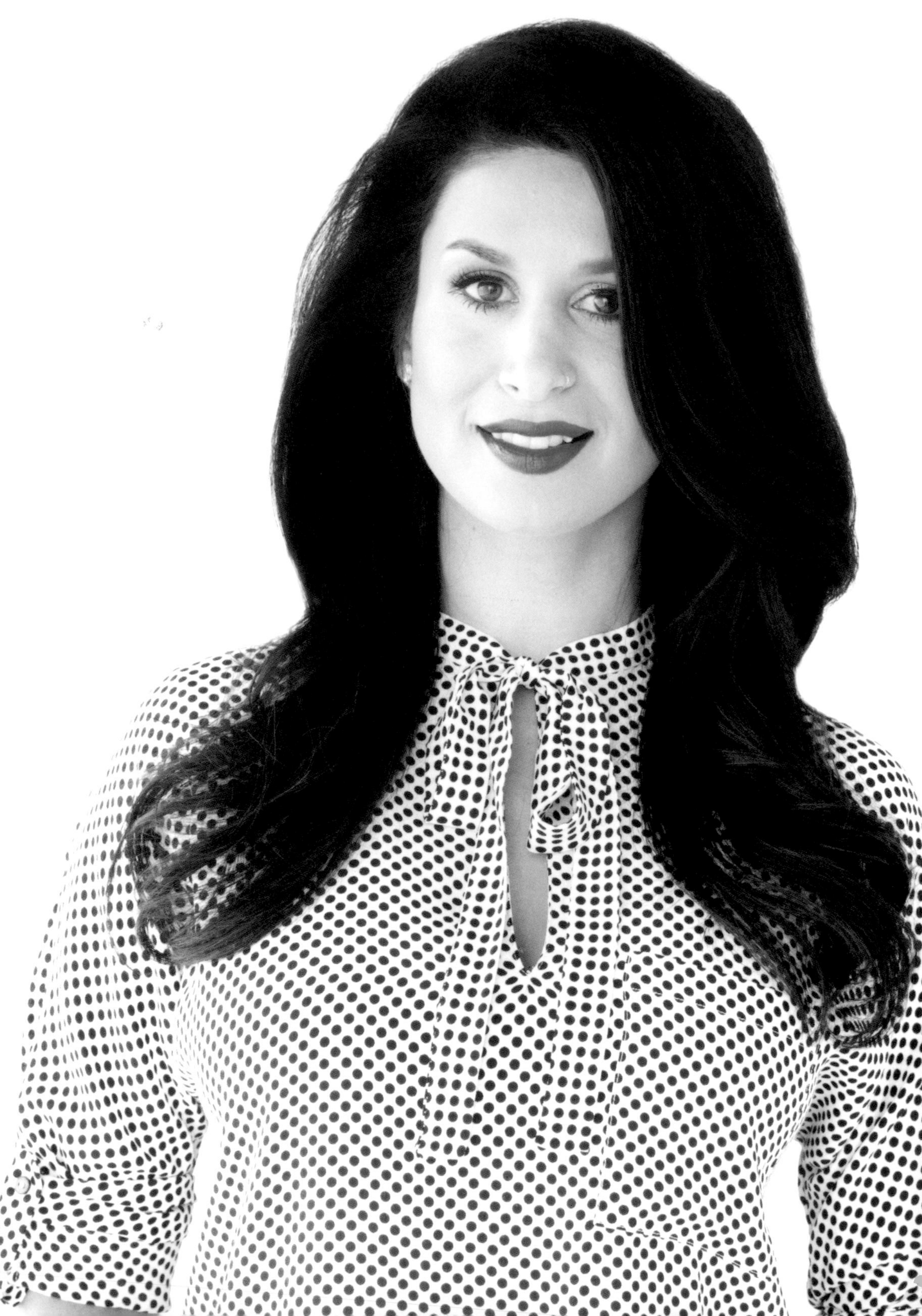

- THE -

SOUTHERN COMFORT

BIG HAIR, LOTS OF VOLUME

PUMP UP THE VOLUME

Ingredients:

Heat protectant

Volumizing mousse

Detangling brush

Blow-dryer

Clips

Medium ceramic-barrel brush

Self-grip rollers

Flexible hold hair spray

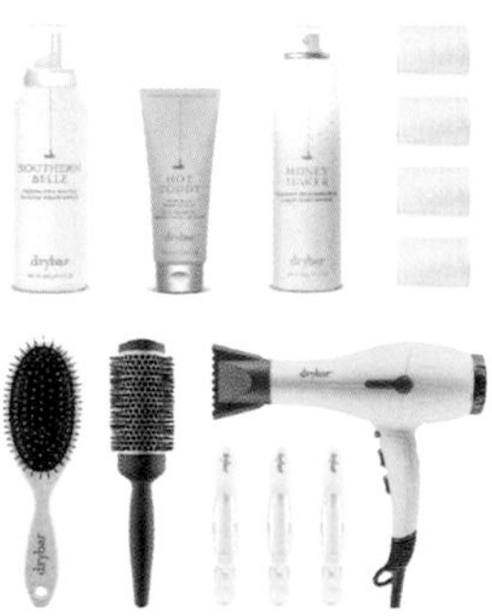

You know what they say: Everything is bigger and sweeter at Drybar (or something like that). This is especially true when it comes to the Southern Comfort, a style for the lady who wants to look done, done, done.

I would like to take a moment to apologize to our short- or fine-haired friends. Unless you're considering adding some major extensions (which is never a bad idea, if you ask me), this look might not be for you. This one goes out to all the women with medium or thick hair that is begging for big, bouncy curls.

One word to the wise: Take your sweet, sweet time. You could dry your hair, set it in Velcro rollers, then sip Arnold Palmers on your porch (or couch) all afternoon. The longer you let this style set, the better off you are.

When it comes to the Southern Comfort, all bets are off.

1. Don't panic. And don't pull your hair into a ponytail, either. Now's not the time. This thick, wavy hair is about to be transformed!

If your hair blows out very easily, go ahead and take out a lot of moisture during your rough-dry. If your hair is prone to frizz, play it safe and leave hair a little more on the damp side.

2. After washing, conditioning and towel-drying your hair, apply a heat protectant like Hot Toddy all over. Scrunch in a marshmallow-size amount of volumizing mousse like Southern Belle at the roots. Brush hair to evenly distribute product. Rough-dry hair, then part and section out the front.

For **extra hold**, dose your volumizing mousse with hair spray before applying to your hair.

Show your hair some extra love! To soften up dry ends, add a hydrating treatment oil like 100 Proof and/or a leave-in conditioner like Mr. Incredible.

If your hair is on the straighter or heavier side, rough-dry less and use products to give it more hold!

If you really love volume, a texturizer at the roots will always give you more, more, more. Spray a few pumps on your hands and rub into your roots to add lift at the crown.

1

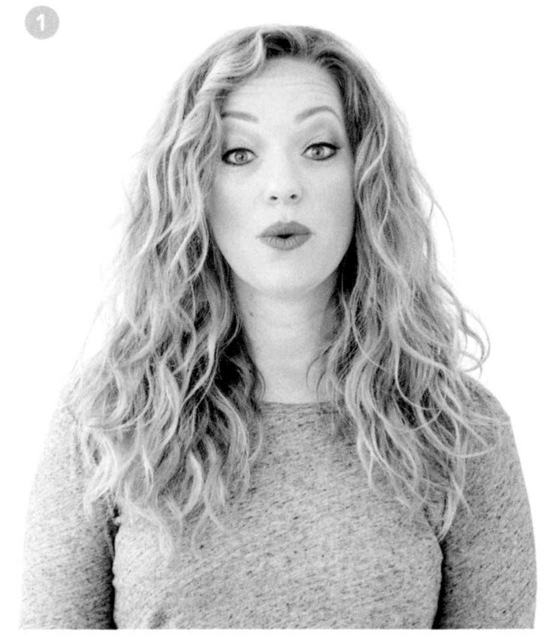

4

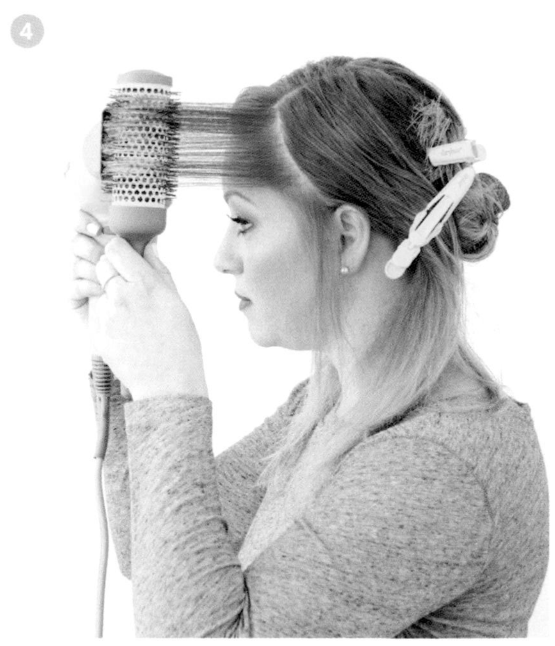

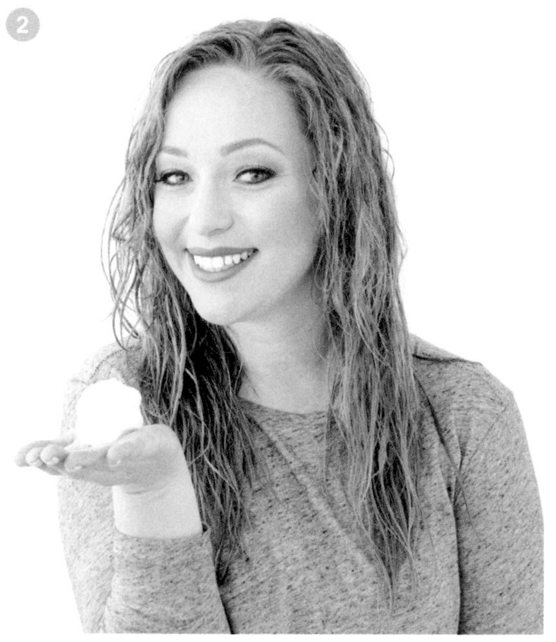

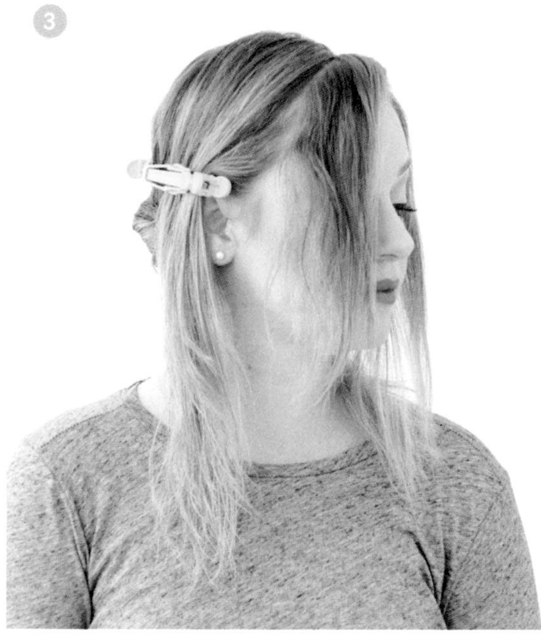

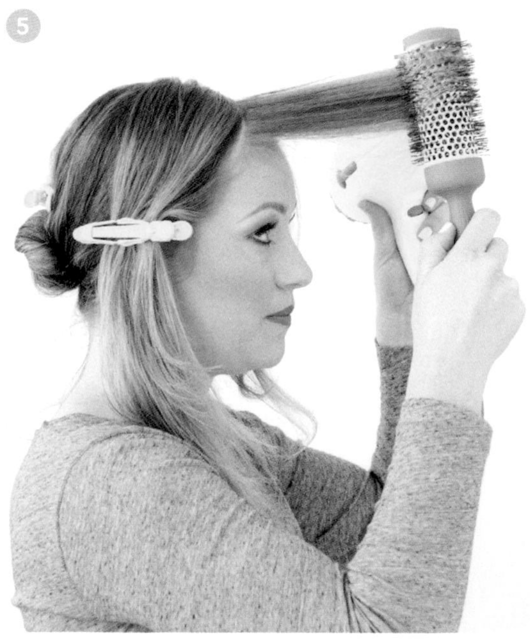

3. Subsection front pieces into manageable 2-inch (5-cm) sections.

4. Using a ceramic-barrel brush like the Half Pint or Full Pint, roll sections vertically from roots to ends to create curl.

5. Work from ear to ear forward, framing your face. A good roll in the brush will give your ends extra shape and bounce.

6. When you twist to release a section from the brush, unwind the hair by spiraling the wrist. This will give you that Farrah Fawcett feathered look (swoon!).

7. To build volume at the crown, start your brush near the roots of a 2-inch (5-cm) horizontal subsection of hair and roll the brush from roots to ends, overdirecting the hair forward.

8. After the section is completely dry, roll down and back from end to roots with a large self-grip roller like a High Top and wiggle into place to secure. Spray the roller with a hair spray like Money Maker to help set the curl.

If you have loads of hair or it's on the **weightier side**, you may want to set the entire crown to ensure good volume and hold. Just go for it!

9. Working in horizontal sections, dry the back of your hair by subsectioning as you work up to the crown.

10. For extra oomph (or if your arms get tired), roll the brush from roots to ends and back again, and leave in place for a few minutes, just like a roller.

11. Once hair has fully cooled, remove the rollers and combine the sections by tousling with fingers.

6

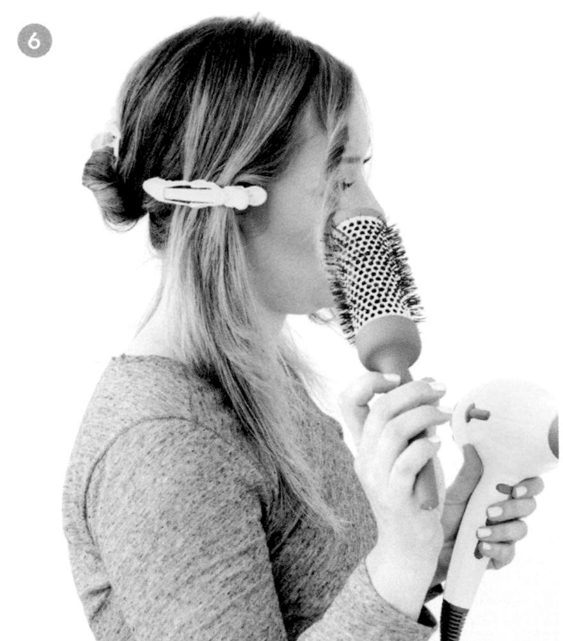

9

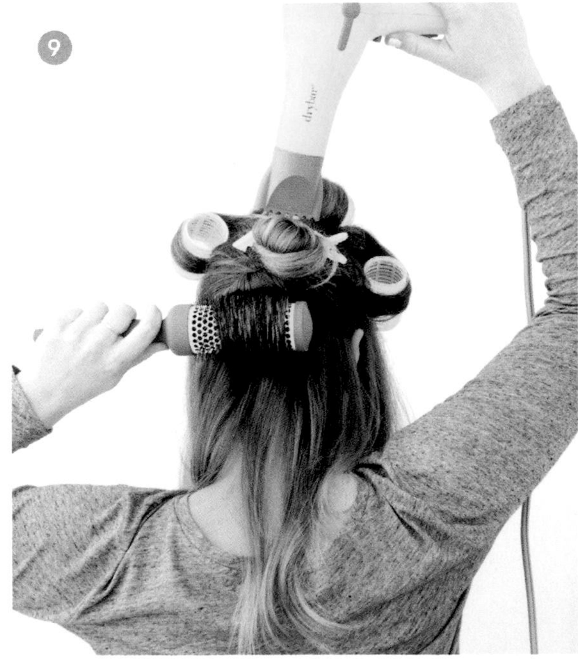

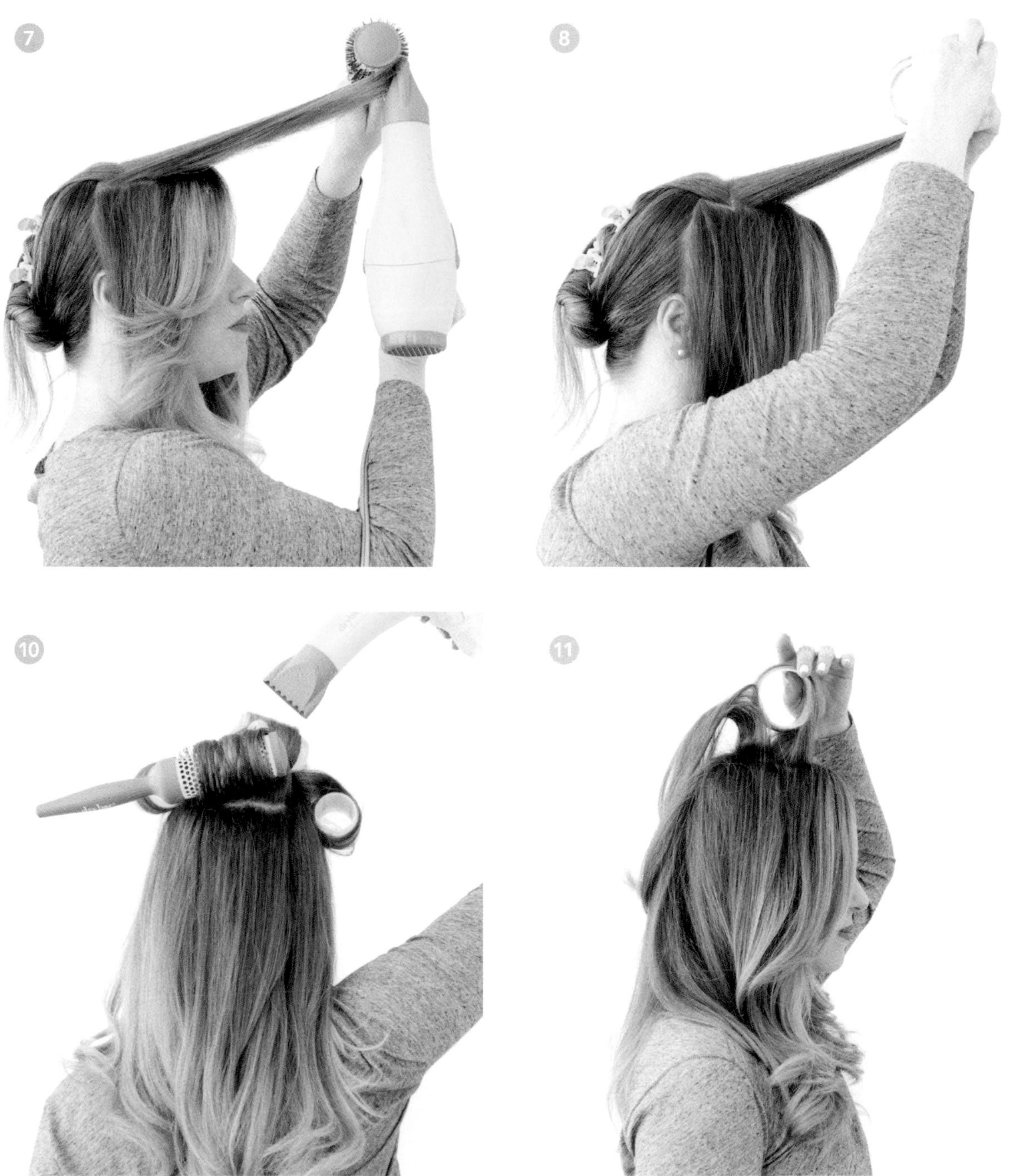
7
8
10
11

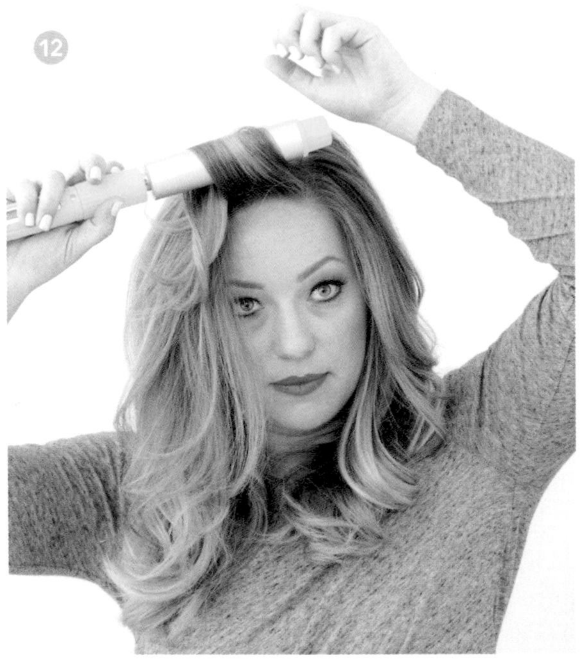
12

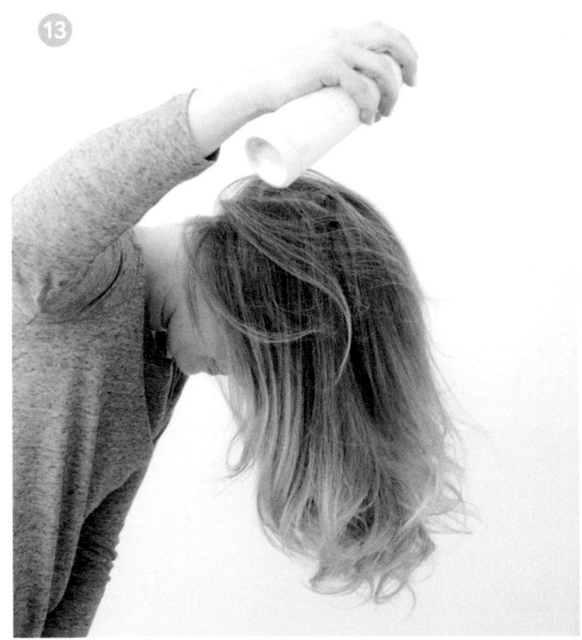
13

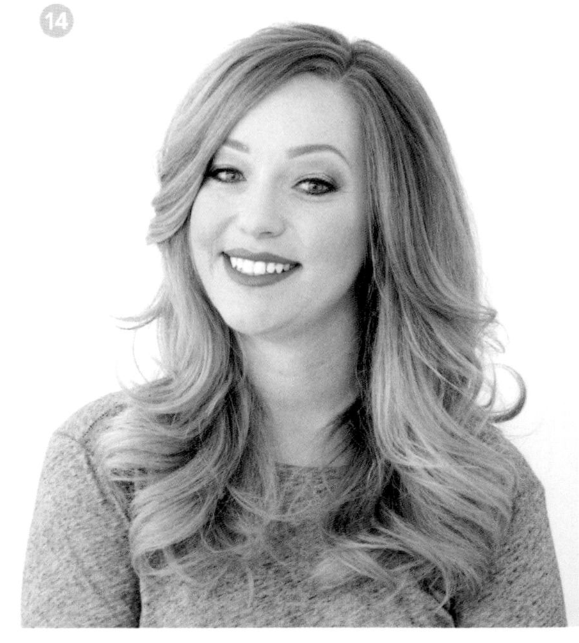
14

12. Why stop now? Going over your curls with a curling iron will smooth the cuticle, erase frizz, and lock in your style. Using a preheated curling iron like the 3-Day Bender, clip in 2-inch-(5-cm-) wide sections of hair at the midshaft; wrap your ends around the wand as you twist the rotating clamp down to your roots. Hold for just a second, then release.

13. Flip hair over and spray with a texturizer like Triple Sec.

14. Once you're right side up, seal the deal with a flexible hold hair spray like Money Maker.

. TIPS .

FOR ROCKING ROLLERS

1. Make sure the hair section is no wider than your roller.

2. Overdirect the section forward.

3. Pull the rollers all the way to the ends so they stay in place.

4. Keep the tension going as you roll hair from ends to roots.

5. Spray with hair spray to set.

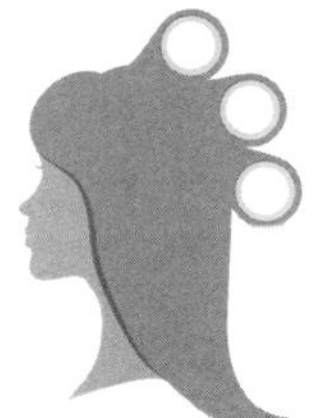

· JUST ROLL WITH IT ·

Even if your ends are a little fried, you can camouflage them by rolling them with a ceramic brush. The hot air from the blow-dryer warms the barrel of the brush and the heat smooths out the cuticle, helping hair look smoother and shiny, ready for more oohs and aahs.

AS DOLLY PARTON ONCE SAID,

"THE BIGGER THE HAIR, THE CLOSER TO GOD."

AND I CAN ATTEST THAT WHEN YOU FINALLY COAX YOUR HAIR INTO A BIG, FULL, VOLUMINOUS SOUTHERN COMFORT,

YOU'RE PRETTY MUCH ALREADY IN HEAVEN.

SECTION 4:

BEYOND THE

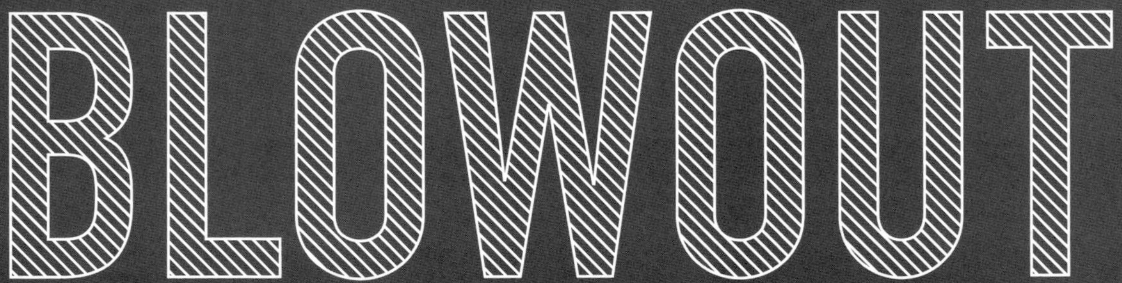

Other Styles to Know and Love

Yes, every day can be a good hair day—but a blow-dryer doesn't have to be part of each and every one.

The perky Perfect Pony, super sweet Fun Bun, and Barmaid Braids are just three of our go-to styles when the Buttercup blow-dryer needs a break. (Hey, even my arms get tired sometimes.)

PERFECT PONY

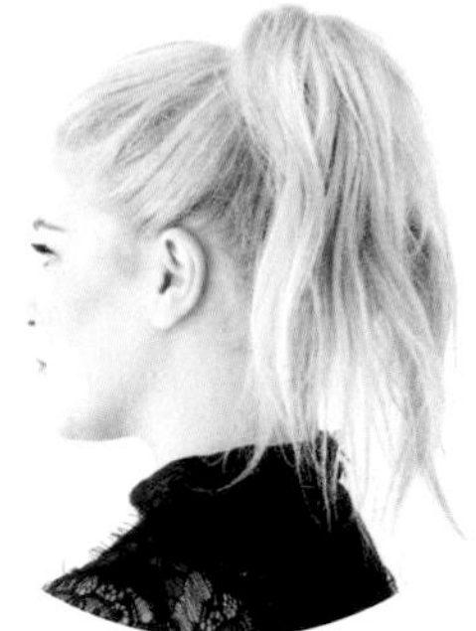

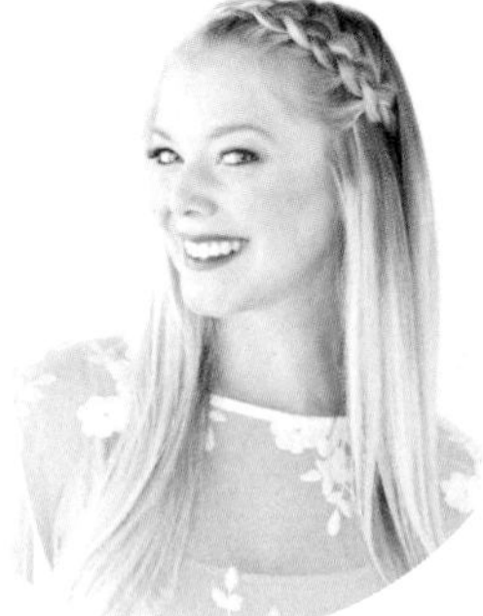

BARMAID BRAID

FUN BUN

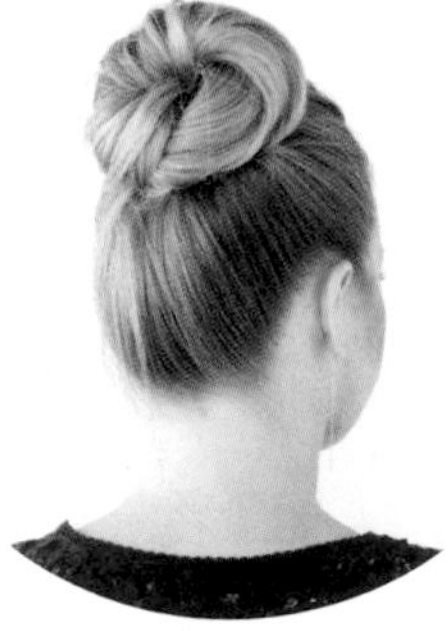

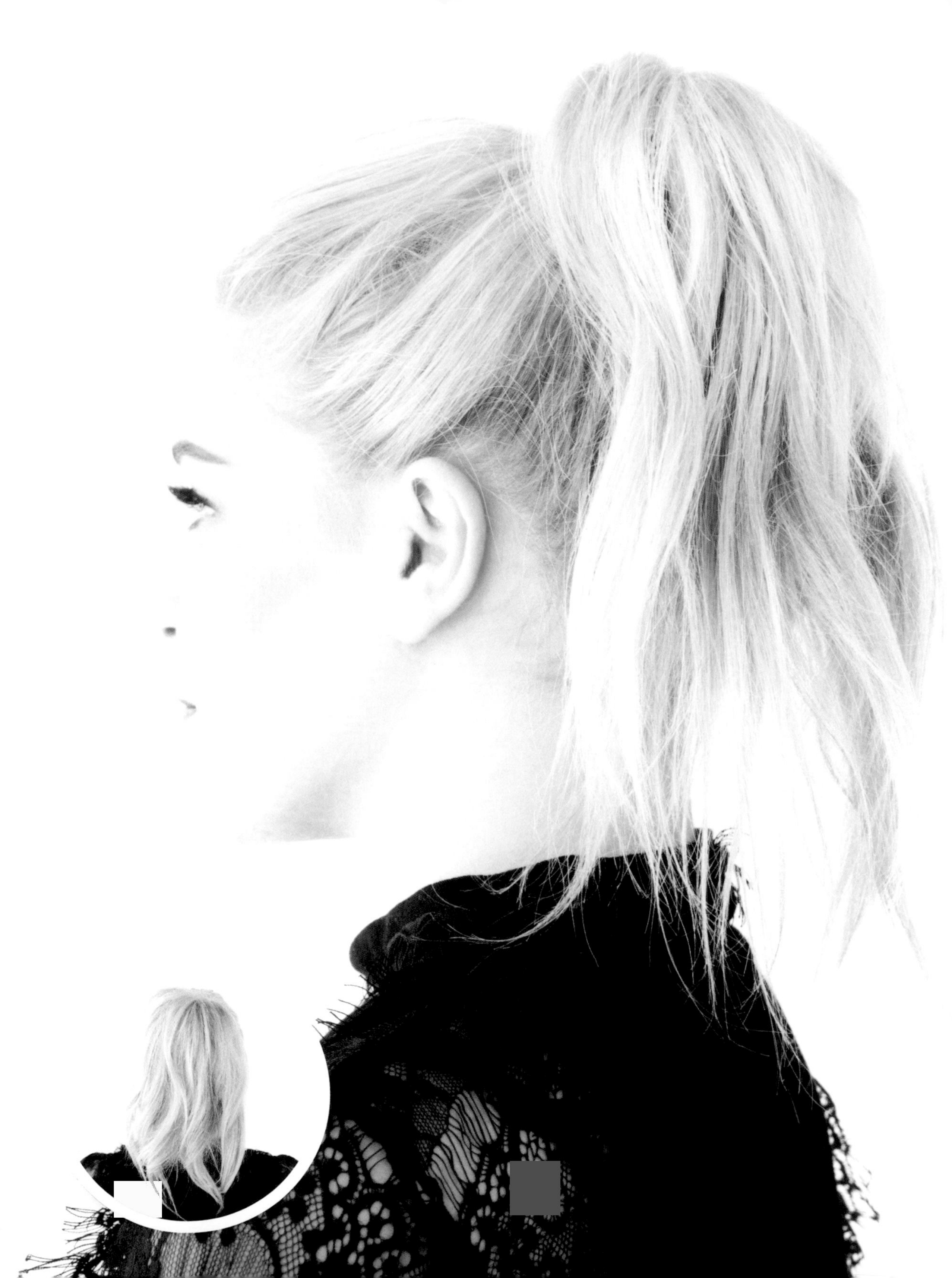

THE
PERFECT PONY

TO THE GYM AND BACK

THE PERFECT PONY

FEELING PERKY?

Ingredients:

Smoothing brush

Clear hair elastic or ponytail holder

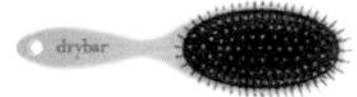

The fastest way to tame a wild mane? A high ponytail.

Often an afterthought or, rather, a last resort, the pony gets kind of a bad rap. But when done well, it's a respectable look in its own right. There're only two things to keep in mind: Make sure hair is nice and smooth all the way around, and give your hair a little volume just behind the hairline and at the base of the pony.

It's the easiest way to pull a look together that I've ever found.

1. It's not the best of hair times, it's not the worst of hair times. It's just that time in between washes when your hair could totally go one more day. Kinda.

2. As you gather all your hair at the crown of your head, use a brush like the Lemon Drop to smooth out major bumps. It doesn't have to be perfect.

3. You can also smooth bumpy hair using your fingers to leave some texture.

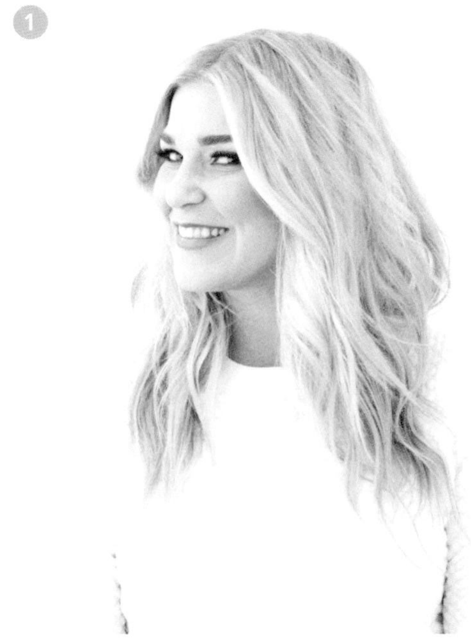

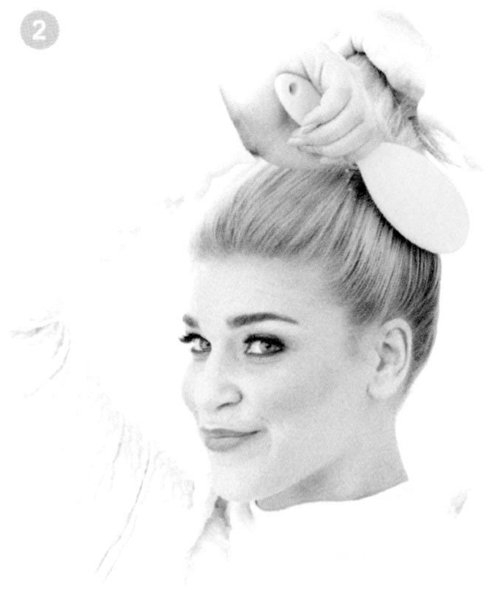

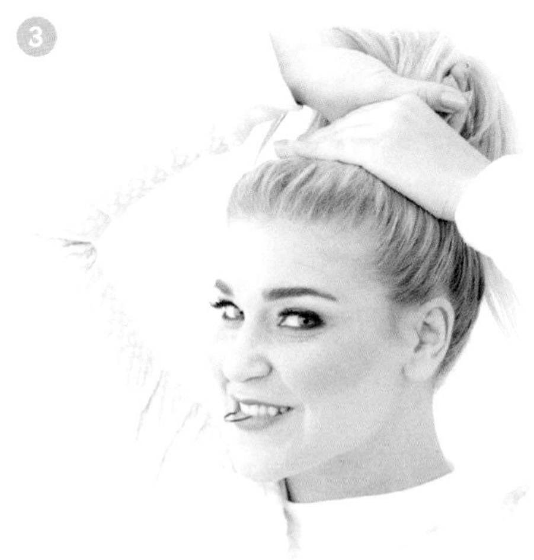

4. Secure the pony at the crown of your head using a clear elastic or a band that is the same color as your hair.
5. Gently tug the hair at the base of the ponytail until it's centered, just high enough on the crown.
6. Run your fingers from your hairline to the crown of your head and pull forward to add a bit of volume.
7. Adjust and pull the ponytail until it's perfectly perky.
8. Tousle the ends, and the pony should be in full swing.

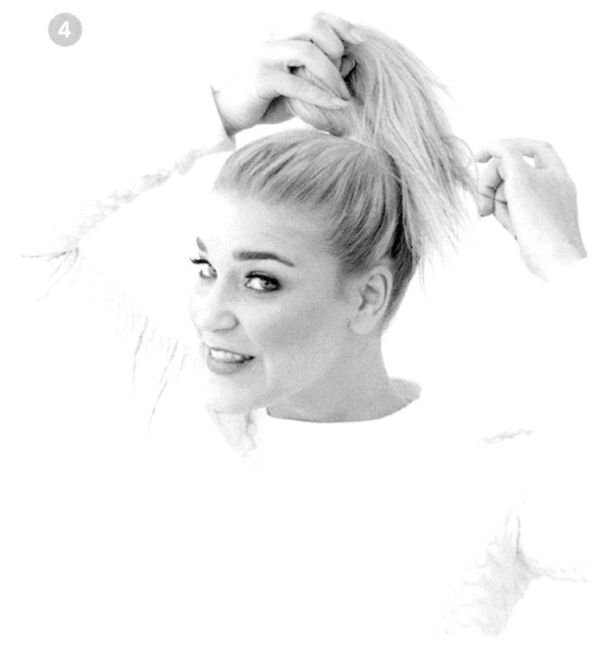

Whoa, Nelly!
Wet hair and tight elastics don't mix. Let hair dry fully before putting it up, and save yourself from breakage.

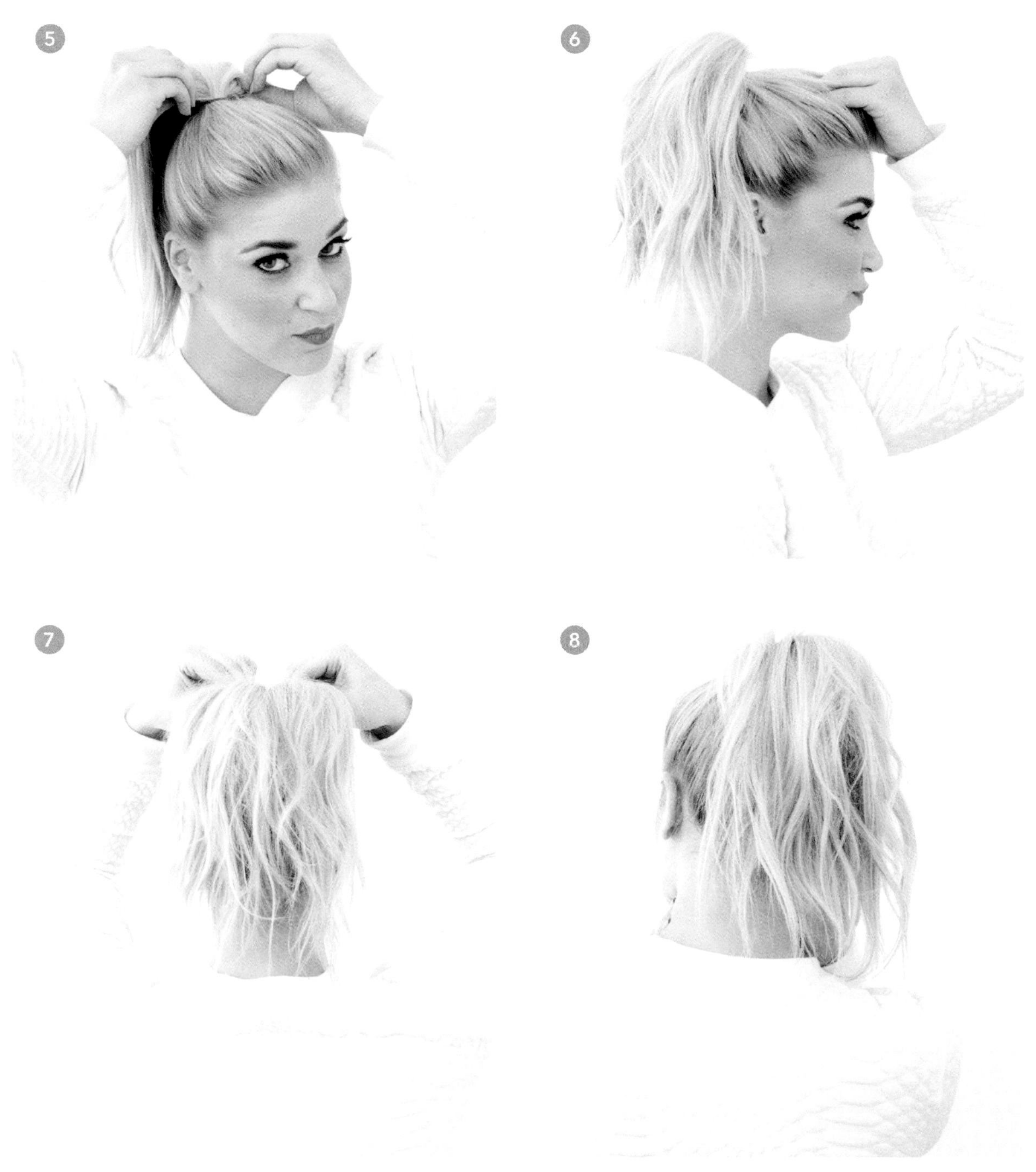
5
6
7
8

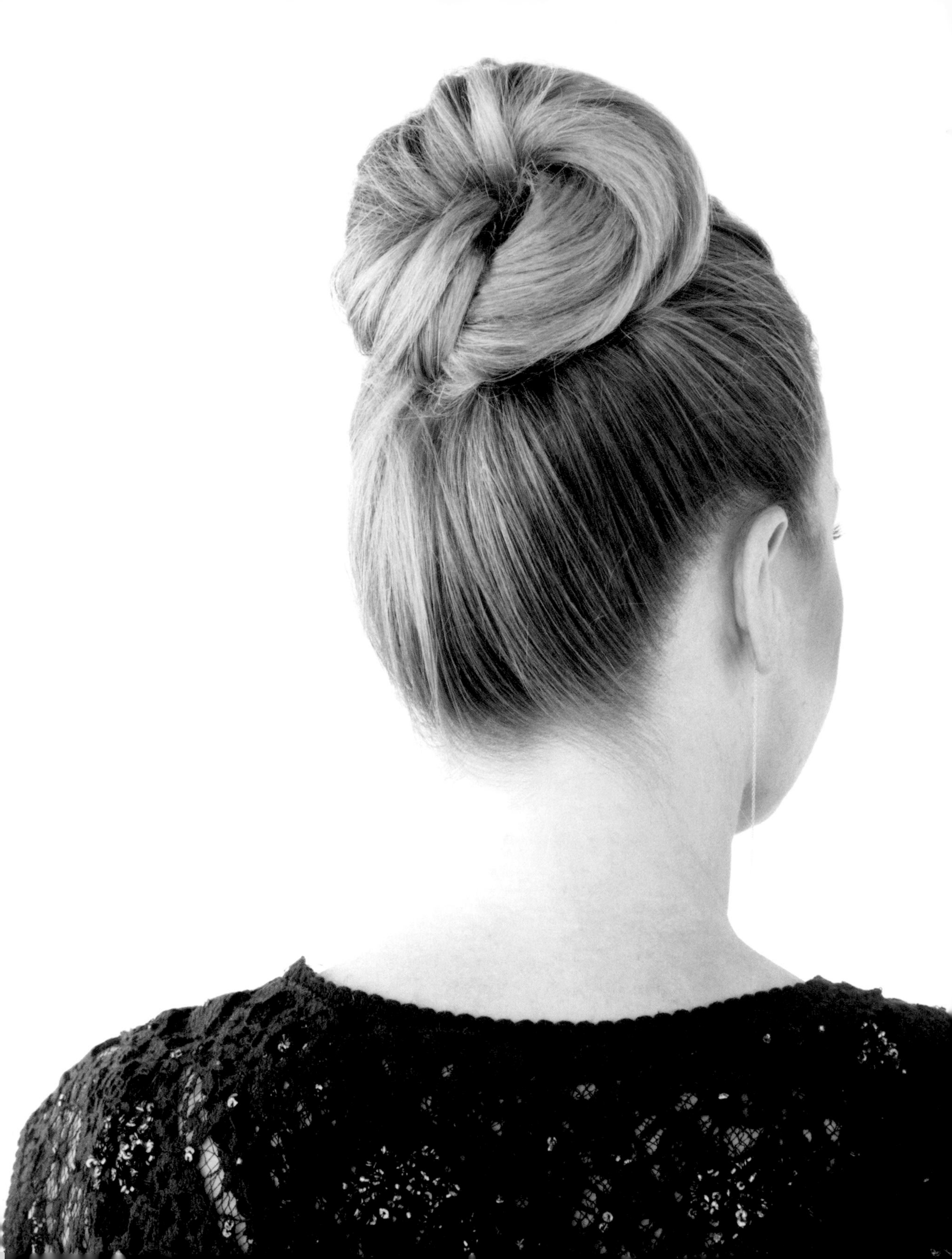

– THE –
FUN BUN

NOT JUST FOR BAD HAIR DAYS

TOP OF THE KNOTS

Ingredients:

Detangling or boar-bristle brush

Clear elastic or ponytail holder

Four to six large bobby pins

Hair spray

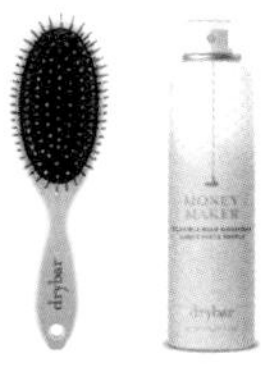

We like to think of the Fun Bun as an instant fix for the bad-hair-day blues. Just saying the words *fun bun* will put a smile on your face. Whatever your hair type, if your hair's long enough to pull into a proper high ponytail, it's long enough for a Fun Bun. A genius option for days when you are pressed for time or your blowout is on its way out, it's easy to master (and still looks good even when it's a touch mussed up).

1. Using your fingers, gather all your hair into a ponytail at the top of your head, high on your crown.

2. Loosely holding your ponytail in one hand, brush hair back to smooth it and remove any bumps.

3. Secure with a clear elastic or ponytail holder.

1

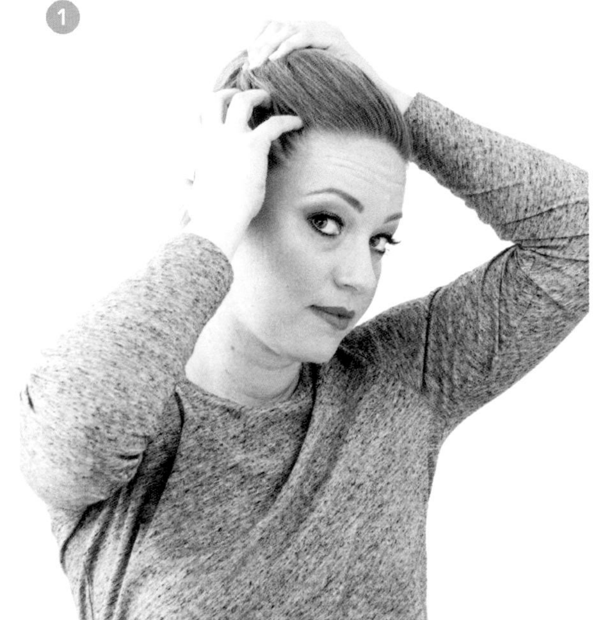

2

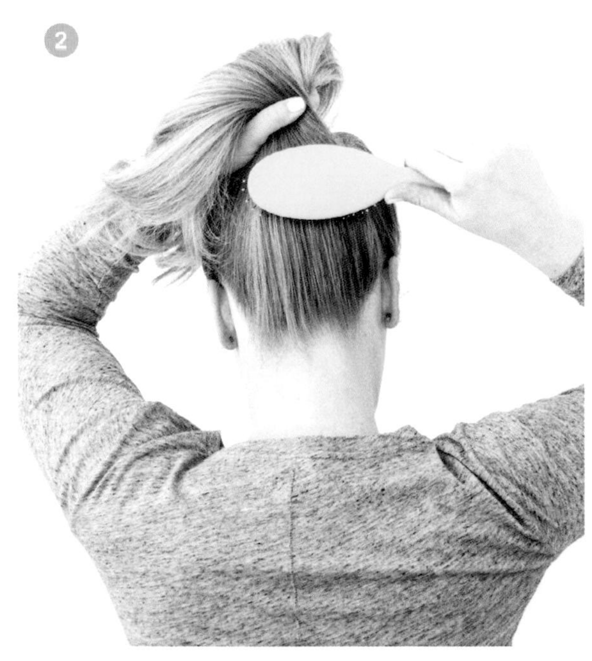

3

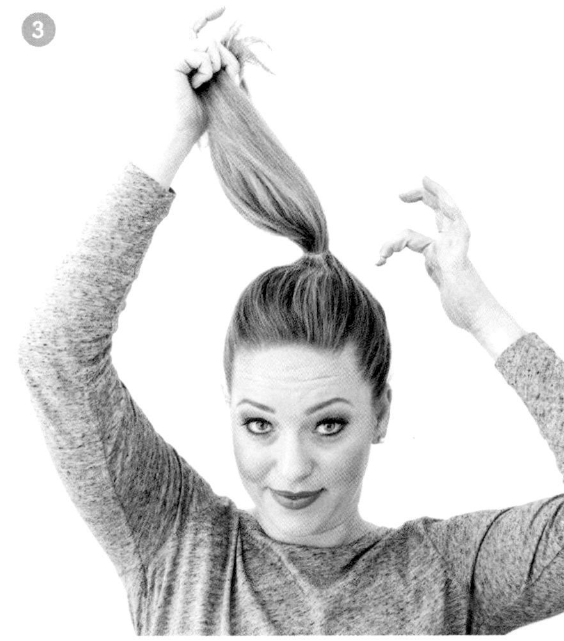

4. Twist hair loosely, then wrap it around the base of the ponytail to shape your bun. Tuck ends under with bobby pins (a girl's best friend).
5. To hold the bun in place, bobby-pin hair around the base as you go.
6. Tuck ends under and pin any loose pieces.
7. Using the palms of your hands, gently smooth flyaways. Spray with hair spray.
8. You're all done. Easy peasy!

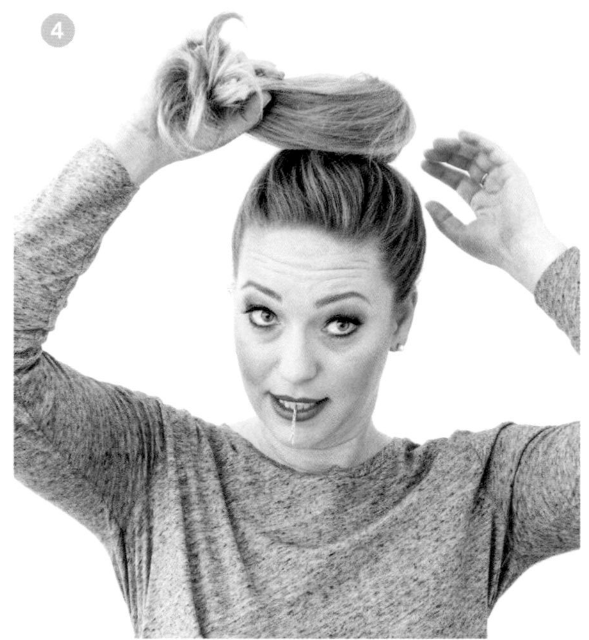

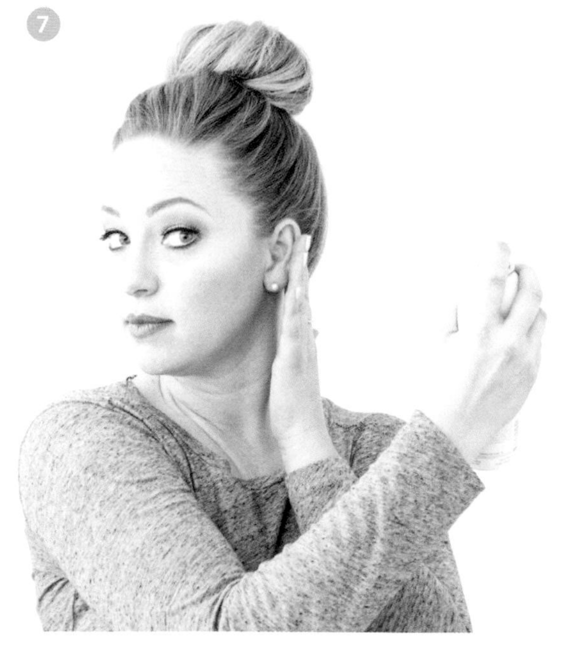

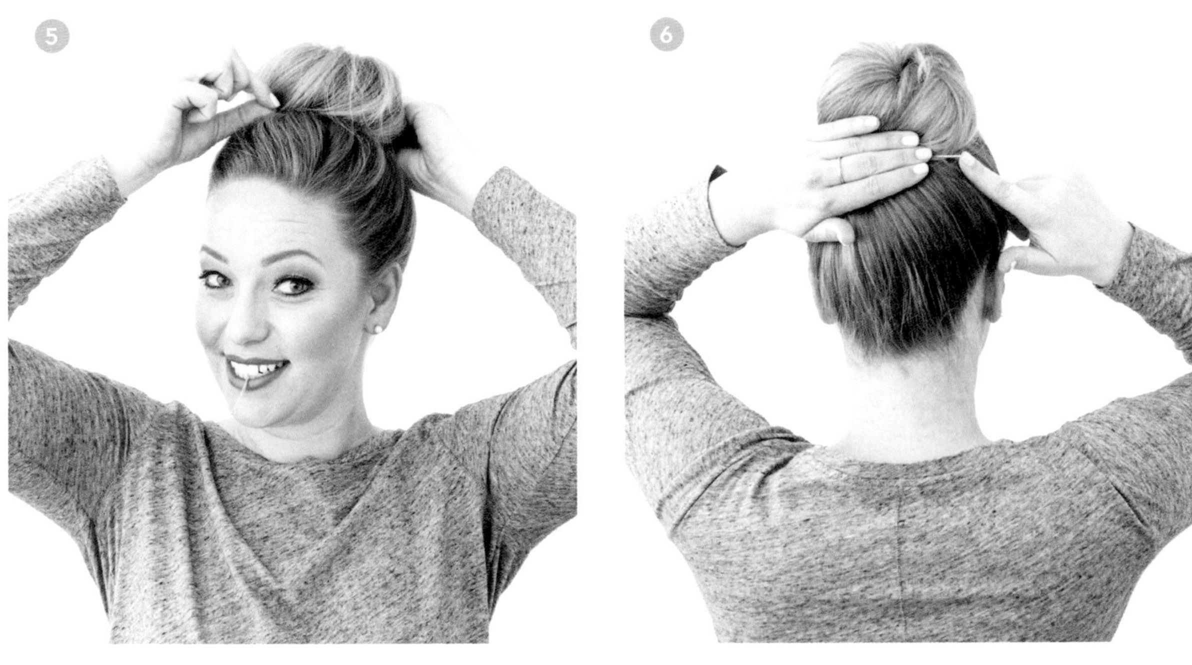
5
6

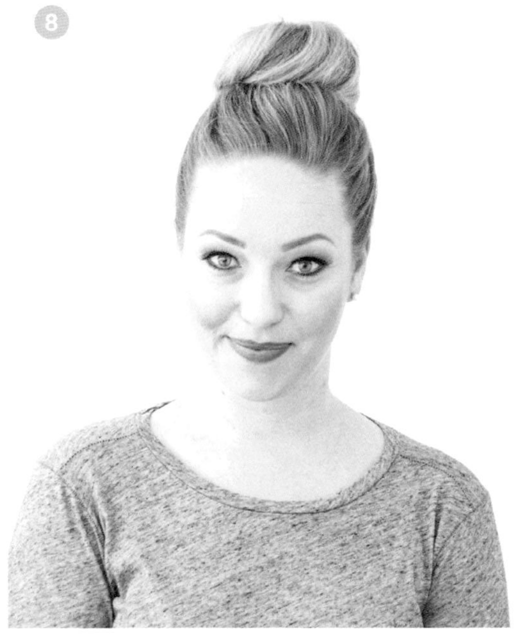
8

- THE -
BARMAID BRAID

AKA WHAT BANGS?

LET'S DO THE TWIST!

Ingredients:

Dry shampoo or volumizing powder

Wide-tooth comb or detangling brush

Clear hair elastic

Bobby pin

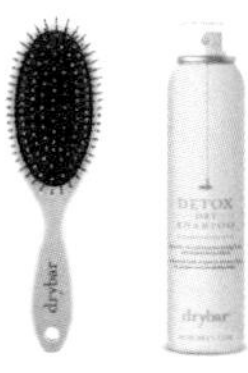

Bangs. Unless it's that one day out of a million when you've woken up and your bangs are just right, it can be a real can't-live-with-them/can't-live-without-them struggle sometimes. For those moments—and all the times when having a braid just seems like a good idea, to mix it up—there's the Barmaid Braid.

Whether your hair is clean or dirty, rubbing a little dry shampoo like Detox or a volumizing powder like High and Mighty in at the roots will create just the right amount of texture you need to make this style last.

1. Starting with dry hair, section out a heavy side part. Choose the side you would normally part your hair on, but go a little deeper. Sprinkle in some volumizing powder or dry shampoo for added grit and texture.

2. Using your side part as your guide, section out a triangle of hair. Split the section into three equal parts. Let's call the section closest to your hairline 1, the middle 2, and the last 3.

3. To braid, 3 goes under 1, then 1 goes under 2. As you repeat this pattern, add hair by pulling diagonal sections from the hairline and the part, and incorporating into each of your three sections.

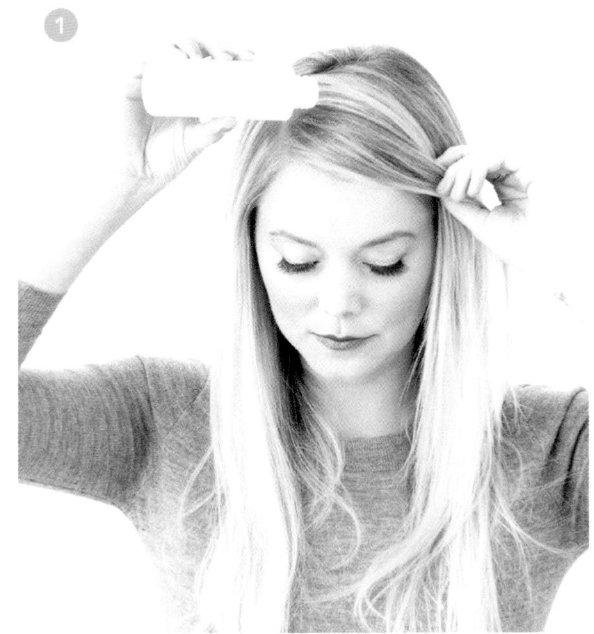

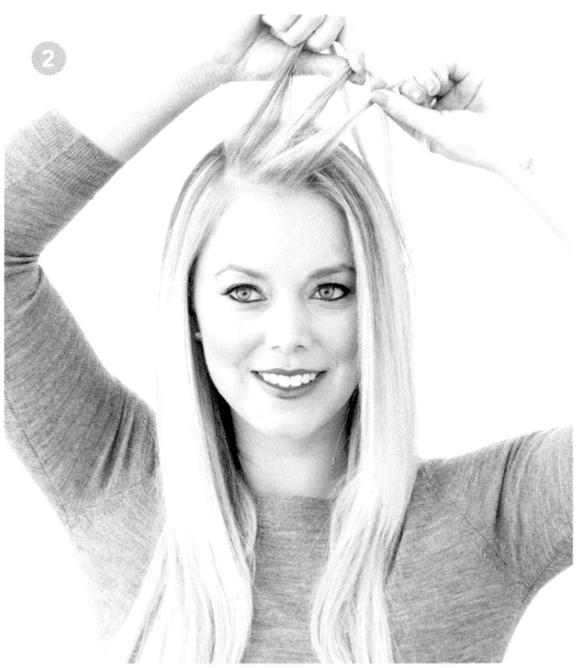

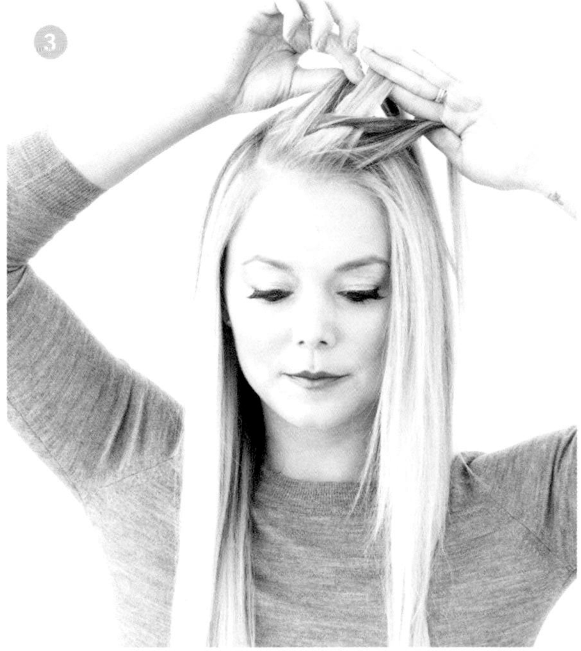

4. Staying closer to the hairline, continue braiding, adding diagonal sections as you go. Easy enough, right?

5. Keep the tension as you go, making sure your braid is even and clean. When you reach your perfect braid length (this is going to be different for everyone), secure with an elastic band. The elastic band should be the same color as your hair, but don't worry if it isn't—it will be hidden away.

6. Now, loosen it up! Starting from the bottom, gently tug the outer loops of the braid to soften the look.

7. Clip the top section of hair behind your ear and secure the braid with a bobby pin in an upward motion. Remove the clip and let the hair fall.

8. For fine-tuning, combine a small amount of shine cream like the Chaser with a short spritz of hair spray like Money Maker, rub palms together, and gently tuck in baby hairs and smooth down flyaways.

4

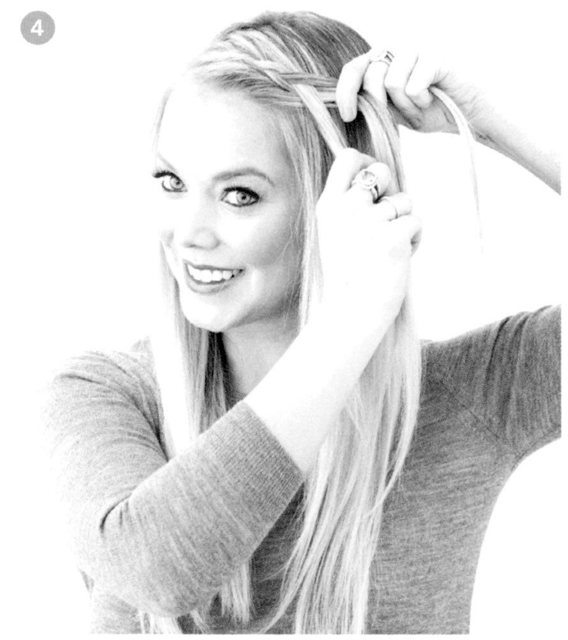

7

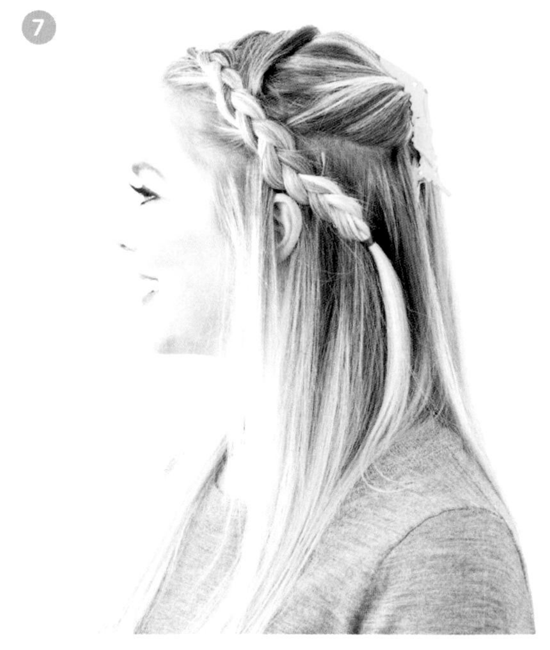

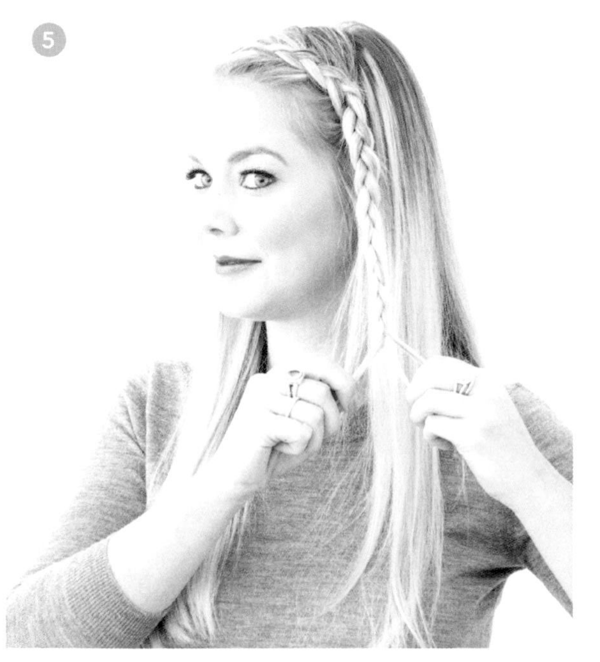
5

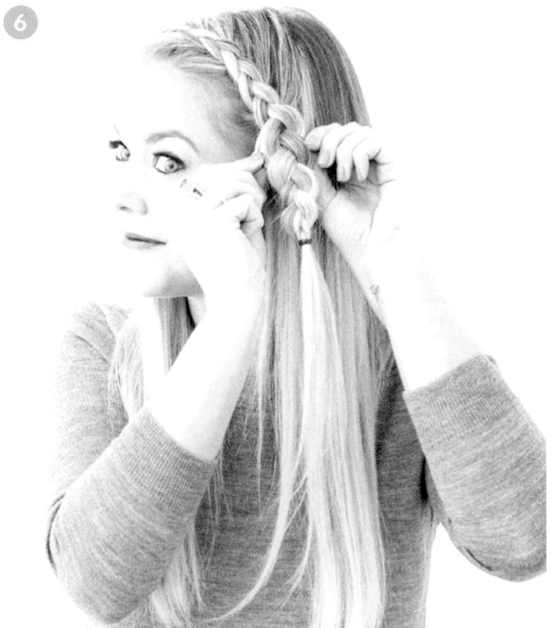
6

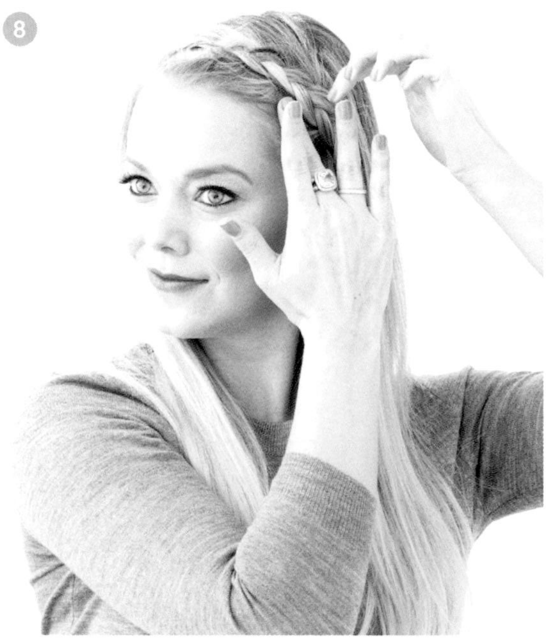
8

SECTION 5:

AFTER PARTY

Making Your Look Last

TOO COOL
Cold weather presents all kinds of special issues, the most annoying of which is definitely static electricity, which can make good hair go bad. To erase damage done by hats and scarves, apply a bit of shine cream to the static area and rub a dryer sheet from midshaft to ends—no joke, it works wonders.

We know nothing lasts forever, not even the perfect blowout. But that doesn't mean we can't try. The good news is that if you've stuck to the Drybar Buttercup Code, then you've already done a bang-up job of setting your style up for greatness. When you start fresh, use the right products in the right way, and pay special attention to smoothing the cuticle down, your hair really should behave for a good few days.

For years (OK, decades) I've been trying everything I can think of to get my blowouts to last for as long as possible. I think my record is a full six days, but that involved very special circumstances and possibly the word *camping*. In real life, I can go three full days before it's braid, topknot, or hat time, but there are plenty of women who say the only time they do their hair (or have their hair done) is at their weekly Drybar appointment (thank you, ladies!).

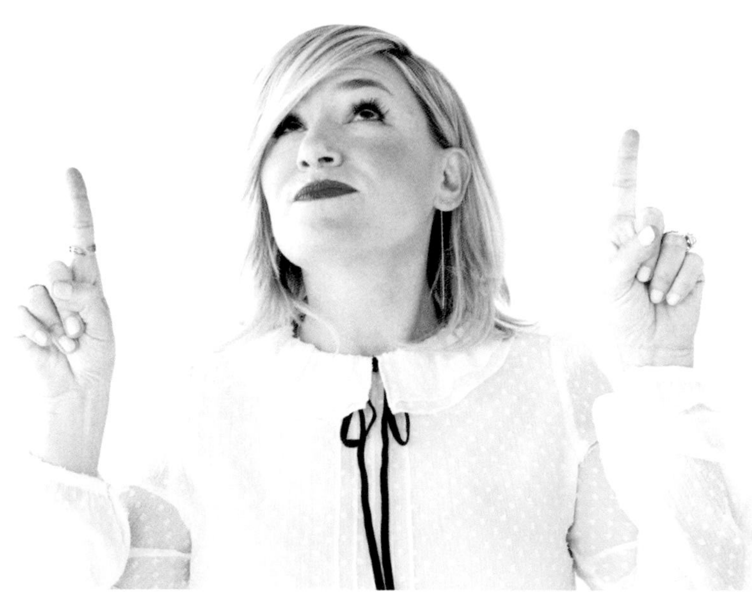

Here are some of my favorite tips and tricks I've collected along the way that I think you should definitely know.

Thinking Cap

One of the best strategies for making your blowout last is to keep your hair as far away from moisture as possible. Since not showering is not an option, a shower cap like the Morning After is clutch. Make sure to tuck in all the fine pieces around your hairline so no water sneaks in. Stick on a shower cap if even you're going to take a bath, since the steam from the hot water can do damage on its own.

Sleeping Beauty

Treat yourself to a silk pillowcase. It sounds like something that would make your grammy very proud, but there are real benefits. Unlike the fibers in a cotton pillowcase, which can rough up the cuticle of your hair and absorb both your natural oils and any products you have used to keep your hair soft and healthy, silk fibers actually help hair maintain moisture and lie smooth, so you wake up with your blowout intact, and way less frizz and friction. It's also very beneficial for your skin. (BTW, I also now sleep in silk pj's, but that's not going to help your blowout. It's just super comfy and makes me feel kinda chic.)

Power Puff

To know dry shampoo is to love dry shampoo. It will save your blowout! The micropowder absorbs dirt, oils, and any odor while giving flat, greasy hair a much-needed boost. Our Drybar Detox dry shampoo is an aerosol spray, so I always give it a good shake, then hold it just a couple of inches away from my scalp and spray one or two quick bursts into my roots. I let it dry for a second, then gently rub it in with my fingertips to make sure it is distributed evenly. In a pinch, I've been known to break out the baby powder. Just tap a little into your palm, rub together with your fingertips, and then apply to your roots. Blend well to make sure there're no white patches left behind!

MAKE SWEAT WORK FOR YOU

A good workout usually means your good hair day is over. Here are three workout-proof styles that work wonders:

So Tai: Pre-workout, gently pull hair into a high ponytail at the crown of your head and twist into a bun; tie it off with a wide, soft hair tie–anything but a hard (sure-to-dent) rubber band–so that you get a wave without the indentation. Post-workout, remove the hair tie, spray in some Detox, tousle, then twist some sweaty pieces, and–poof!–you've got yourself a Southern Comfort mixed with a Mai Tai.

Not So Tai: Pre-workout, pull hair back into a low ponytail (or two) at the nape of your neck, twist hair tightly, and wrap into a low bun; secure with a wide hair tie (no hard rubber bands, please!). Post-workout, remove the hair tie and loosen curls, twist and add some Triple Sec three-in-one texturizer, and–voilà!–it's a quickie Cosmo-Tai.

Virgin Tai: Pre-workout, draw hair in the middle and divide into two sections. Loosely braid each section until there are 1 or 2 inches (2.5 to 5 cm) left at the ends. Secure with a soft hair elastic. Post-workout, remove elastic, shake out the braids, and–ta-da!–it's a mini Mai Tai.

If you are hitting the shower after your sweat sesh, take out your hair tie before you slip on a shower cap. The steam from the shower will help soften any of the hard bends or indentations that the hair tie may have left.

No time to rinse? Hit hair with the dryer after your workout to remove any left over moisture. The nano-ionic technology blasts out odor and helps re-seal the hair shaft.

AVOID, AVOID, AVOID

BLOW-DRY BUSTERS

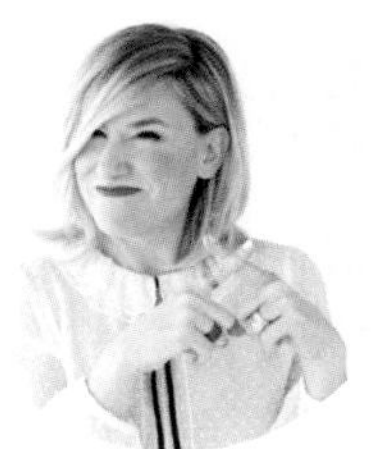

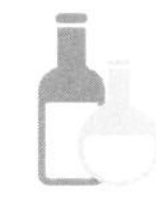

Oil massages

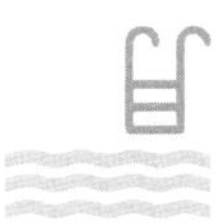

Swimming

Overdoing it with the shine serum

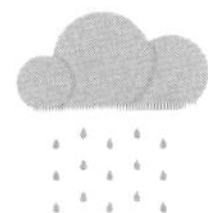

Getting caught in the rain

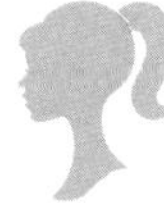

Super tight ponytails

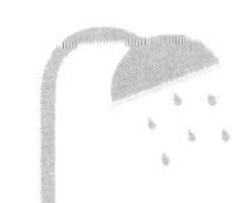

Showering without a shower cap

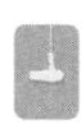

Not rinsing conditioner completely out in the shower

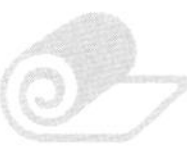

Hot yoga

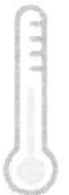

Steaming in a sauna

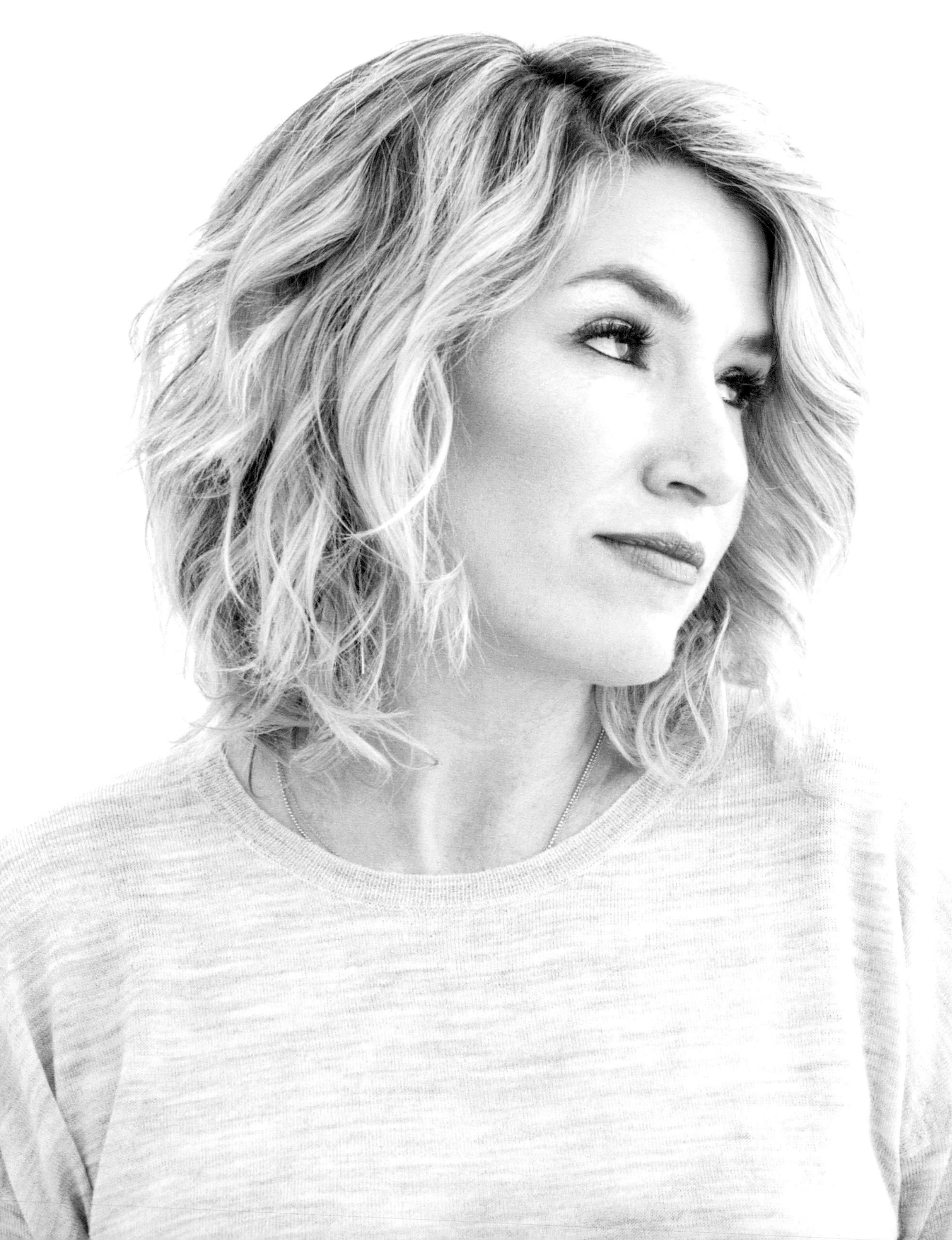

– THE –
DRY TAI

THE MAI TAI IN A MINUTE

THE DRY TAI

TAI ONE ON

Ingredients:

Clips

Curling Iron

Volumizing or texturizing spray

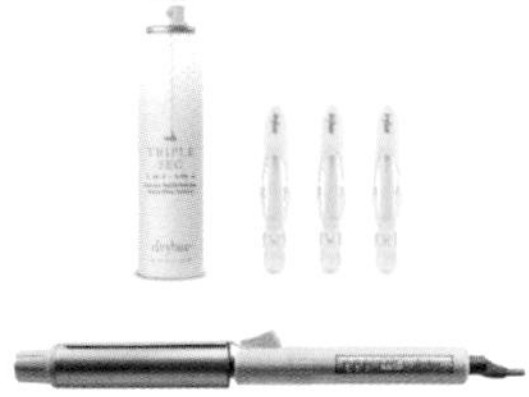

For those days when you skipped the blowdry but suddenly have a ________________ (fill in the blank with that super exciting thing that you're really stoked to do) and only a few minutes to get out the door, meet the Dry Tai, a take on the Mai Tai (hold the blow-dryer).

1. Here, I present the I-skipped-my-blow-dry-'cause-I-thought-we-were-gonna-watch-*Clueless*-on-the-couch-but-now-we're-going-out look. D'oh!

2. Starting in the front, section out bangs and clip the rest of your hair back and out of the way. Using a preheated curling iron, grab 1- or 2-inch (2.5- or 5-cm) sections of hair and curl pieces away from your face.

3. Moving along your part, continue curling sections around your head.

1

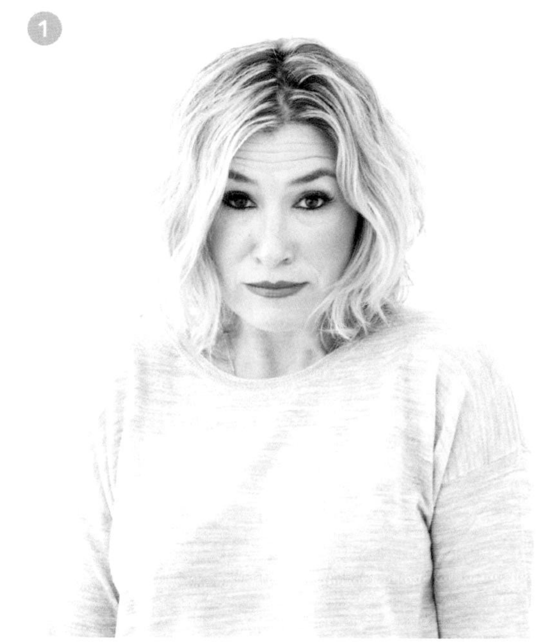

2

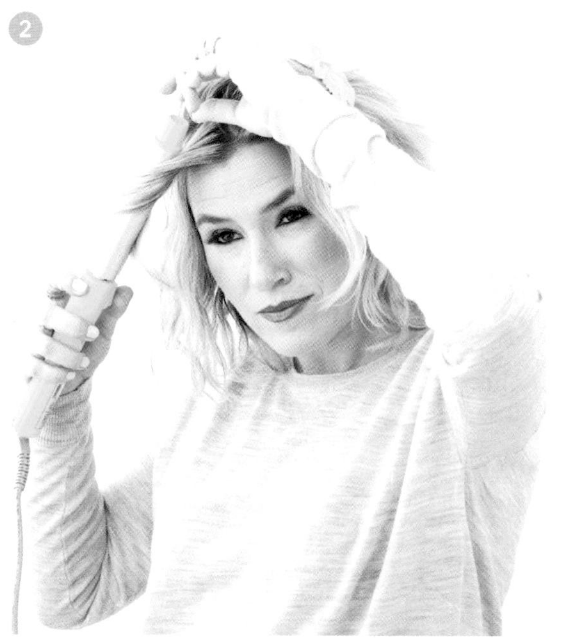

3

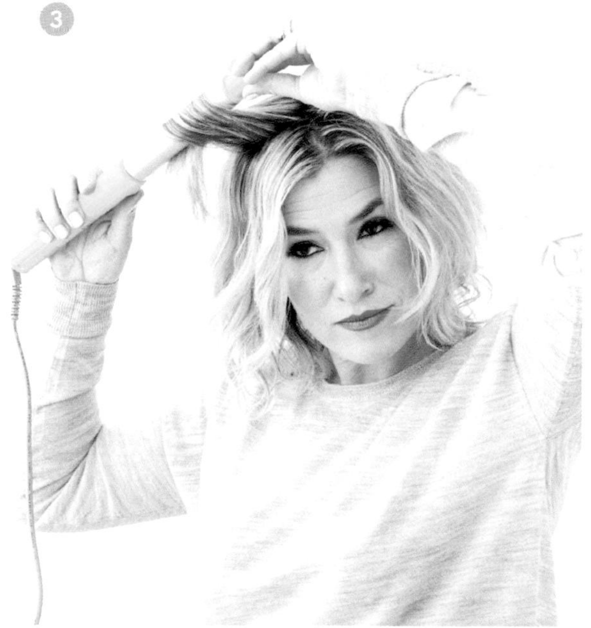

4. Section off the top half of your hair and continue curling away from your face, just as you did on the other side.
5. Release the top section, letting the rest of the hair down, and finish curling.
6. Alternate the direction of the curl for more texture and movement.
7. For even more texture and volume, lift hair, spray underneath with a volumizing spray, and tousle.
8. And just like that, you're ready to run out the door.

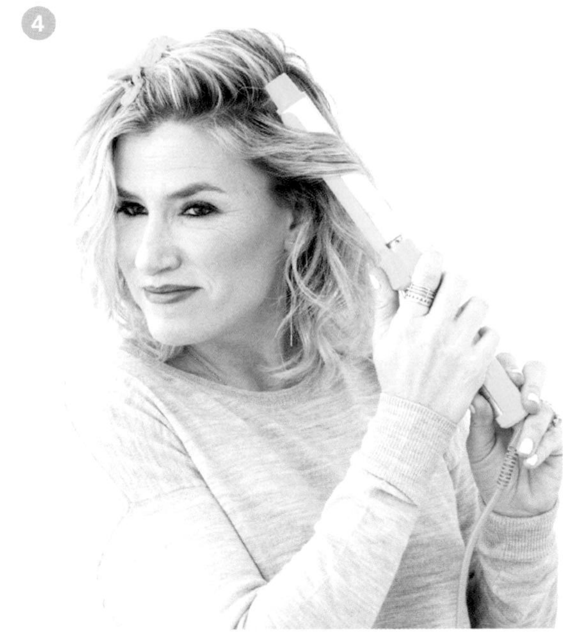

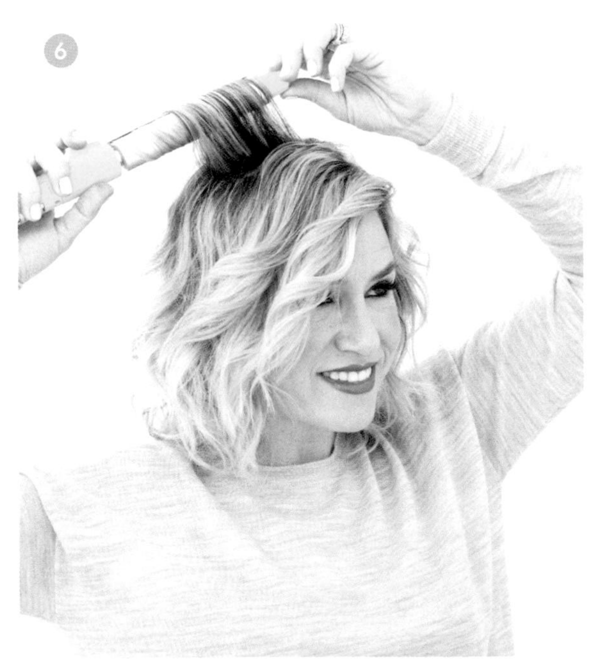

Look Ma! No Clips!
It might look like I'm breaking all the rules here, but when you've been doing this as long as I have, sometimes you just wing it. The finished look isn't as polished as it would be if you followed the step-by-step to a T, but nobody said hair had to be perfect to be pretty.

5

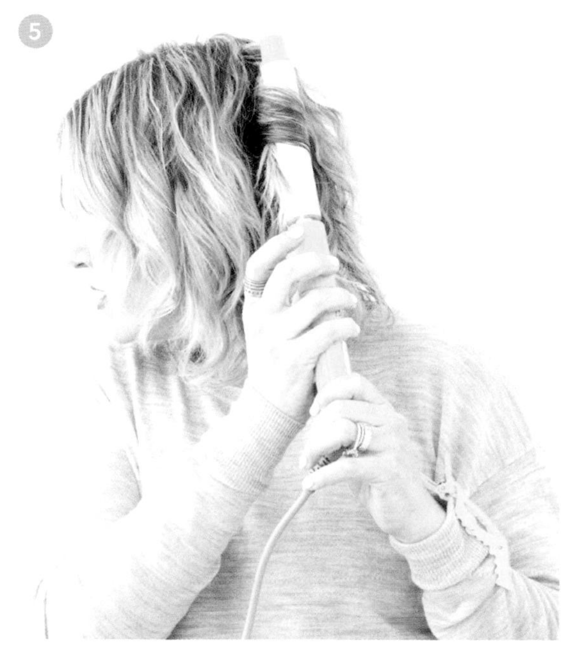

7

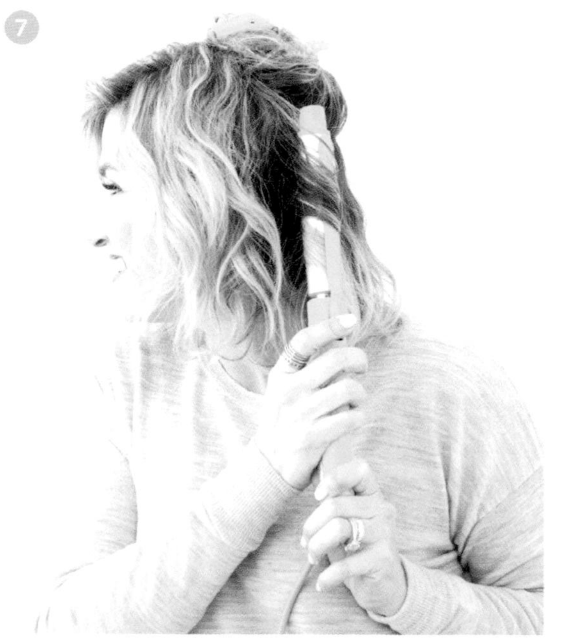

8

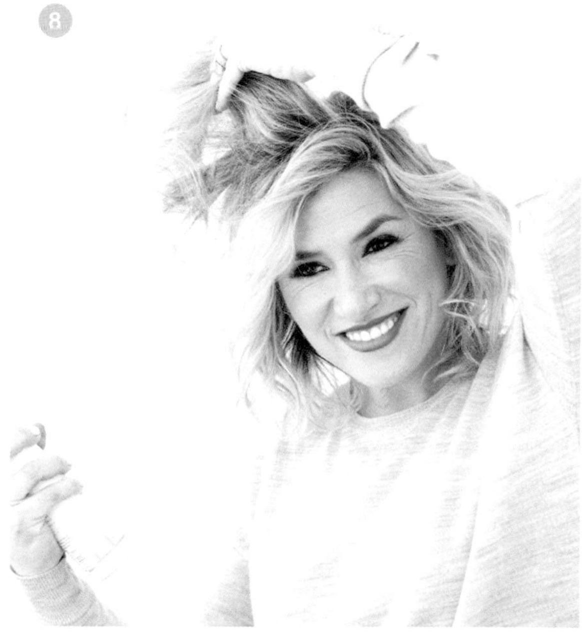

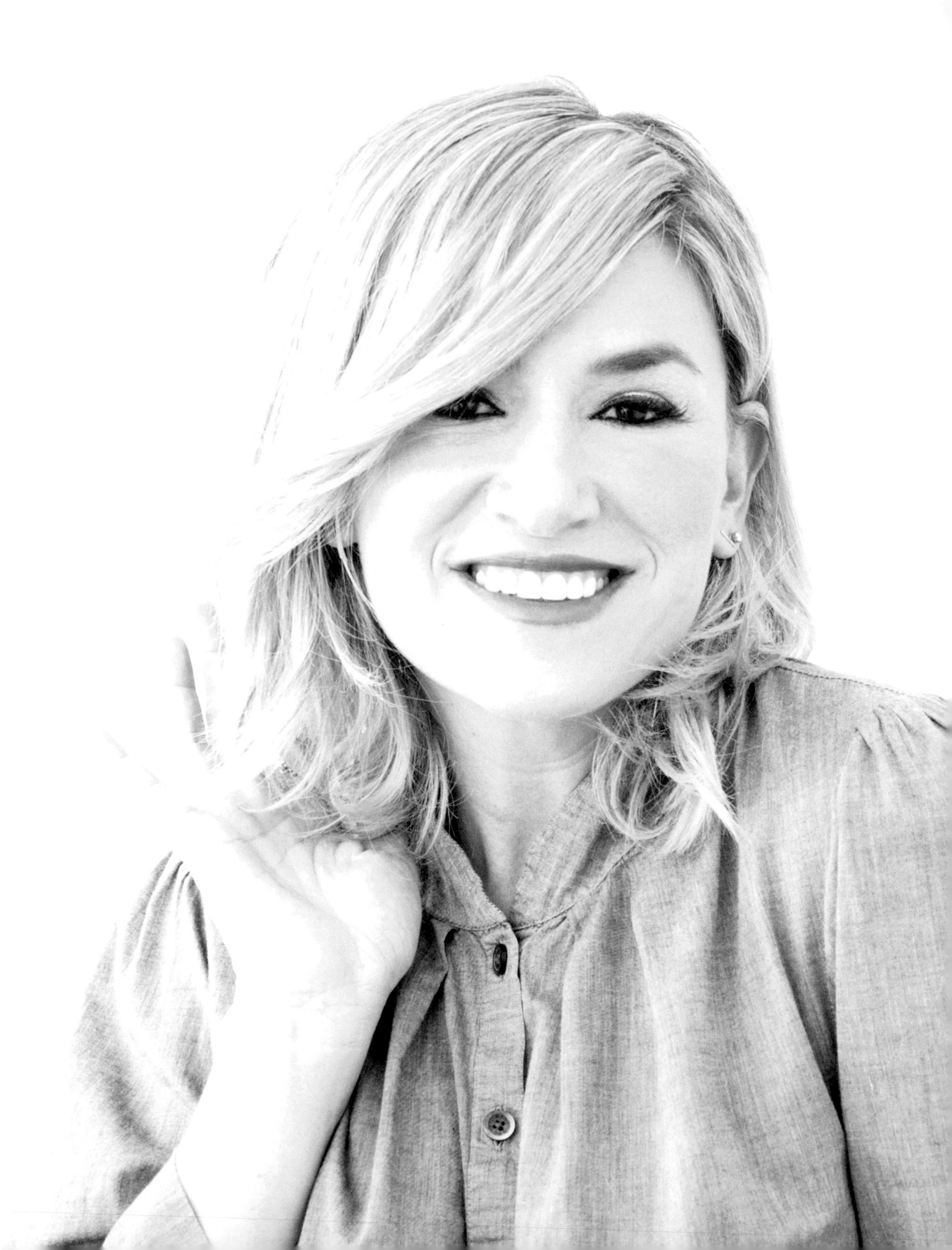

– THE –
STRAIGHTER UP

SECOND-DAY HAIR, SERVED NEAT

THE STRAIGHTER UP

SO NICE, WE STYLED IT TWICE

Ingredients:

Heat protectant or priming mist or spray bottle with water

Medium ceramic-barrel brush

Blow dryer

Dry shampoo

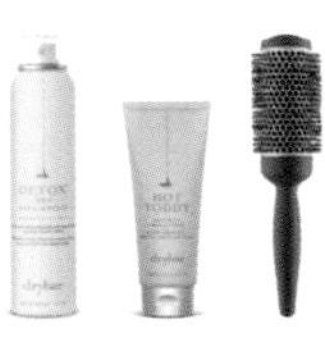

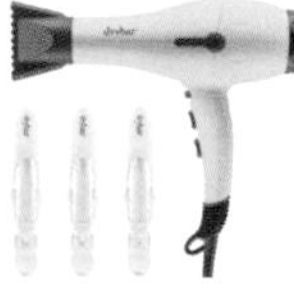

Sometimes all it takes to hit the refresh button on your style is a few seconds of quality time with your dryer and a brush.

1. Your blowout has seen better days—like, say, yesterday (or the day before)—but you're not quite ready to give up on it yet. Don't fret. In less than ten minutes, you can revive your look.

2. Section out the hair you want to work with and clip the rest out of the way, then spritz your hair with a bit of heat protectant and/or primer before re-blow-drying. If you don't have that handy, use a spray bottle filled with water to dampen hair. More than that and you might as well start over.

1

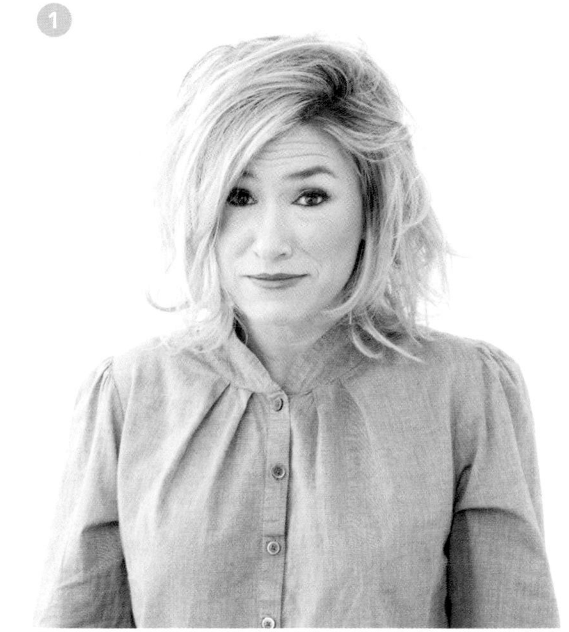

2

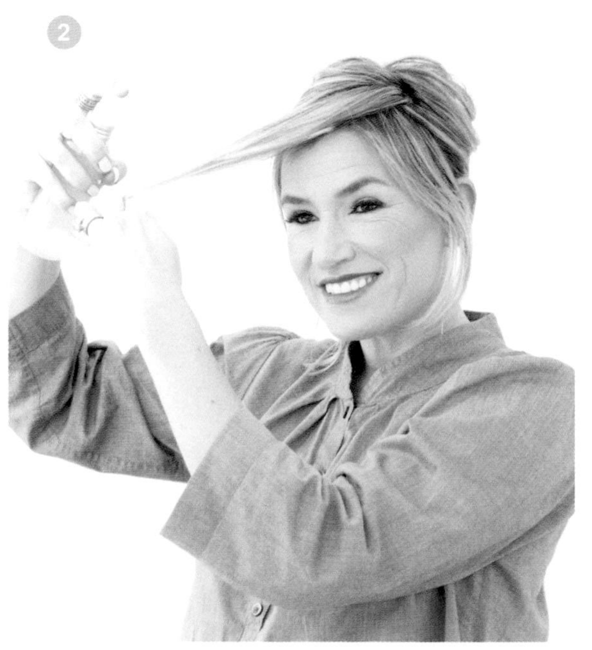

Never, ever blow-dry hair that is already dry. (Pinky swear!) That's a recipe for disaster.

3. Using a small or medium round barrel brush (smaller brush, more curl; medium brush, less curl), blow bangs dry by picking up a horizontal section from your part and roll the brush from roots to ends forward and away from your face. Release the ends with a twist of the wrist and let hair cool and set.

4. Once you're finished in the front, rebuild a bit of volume at the crown. Take a 2-inch- (5-cm-) wide section and roll it from roots to ends and back again.

5. Freshen up a few pieces in the back, and the ends, by repeating steps 2 and 3.

6. A few bursts of dry shampoo will absorb excess oils and add body.

7. Concentrate at the roots to add lift to roots that need a boost and leave hair feeling (and, um, smelling) fresh and clean.

8. Sometimes second-day hair looks even better than the first time around.

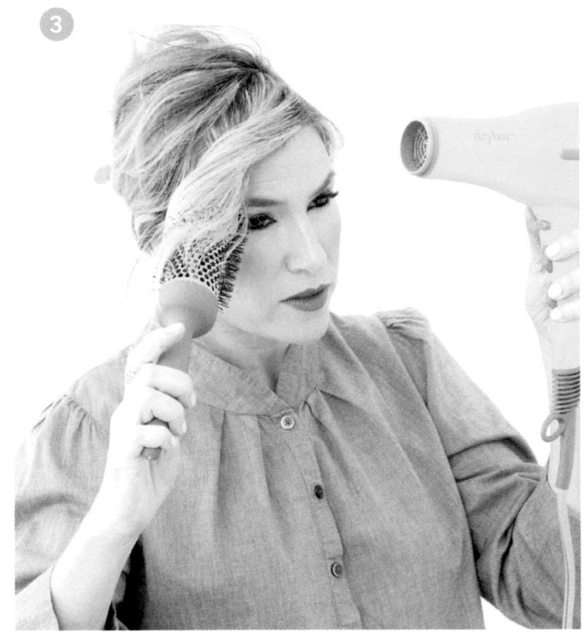

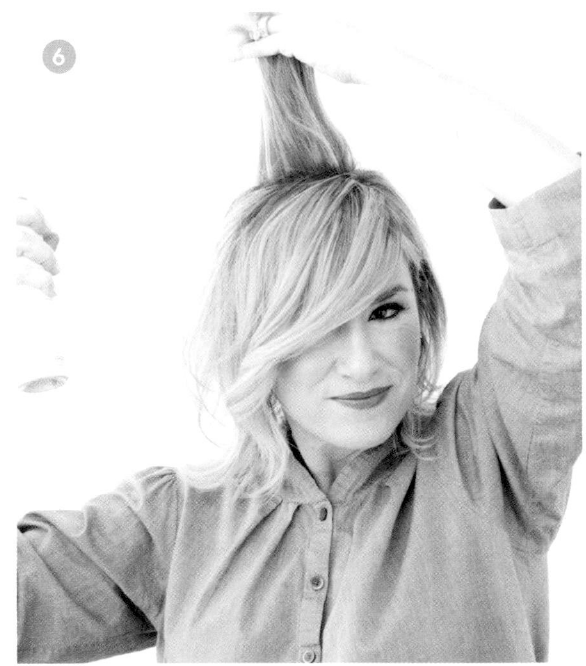

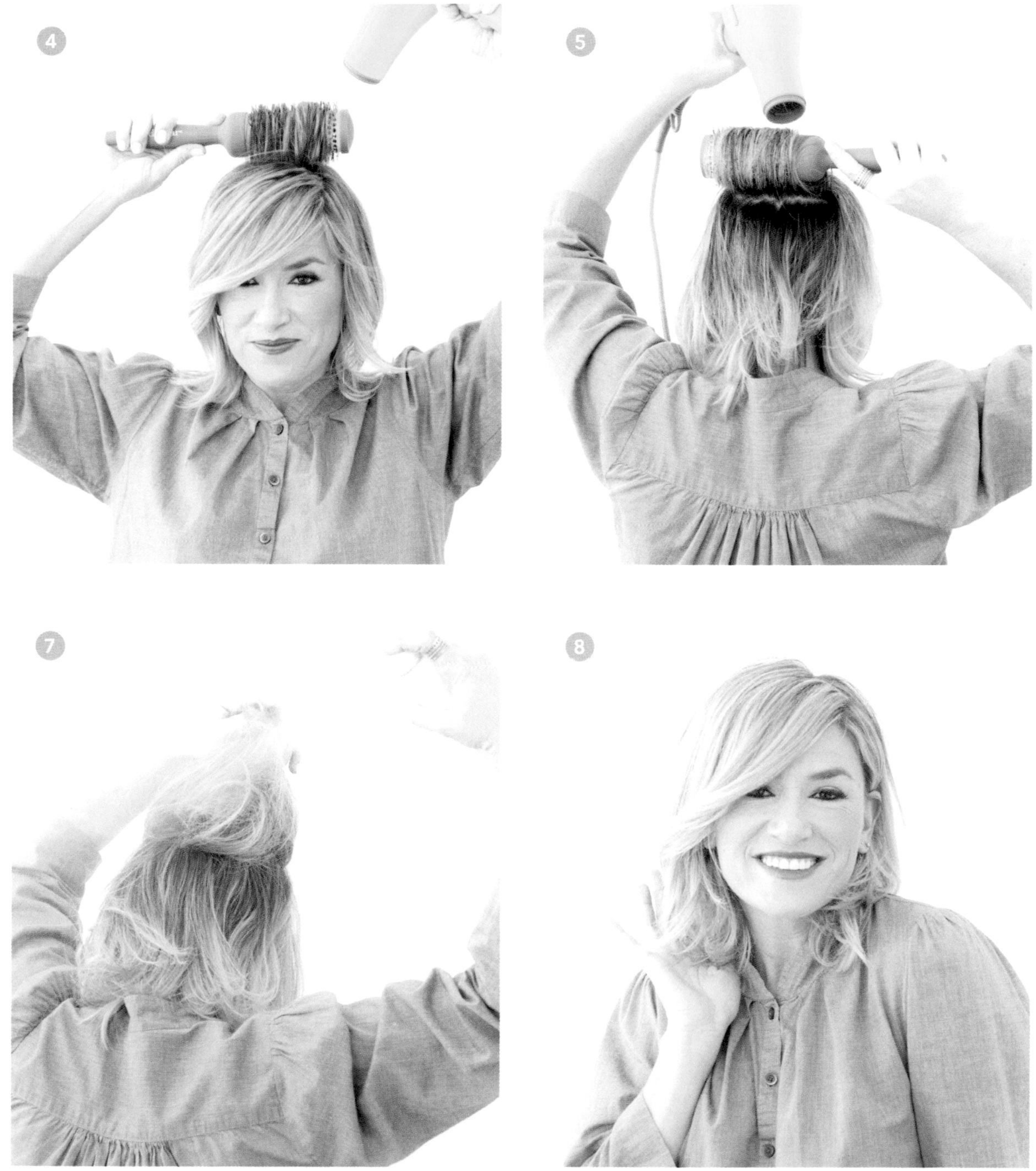
4
5
7
8

SECTION 6:

Q & A

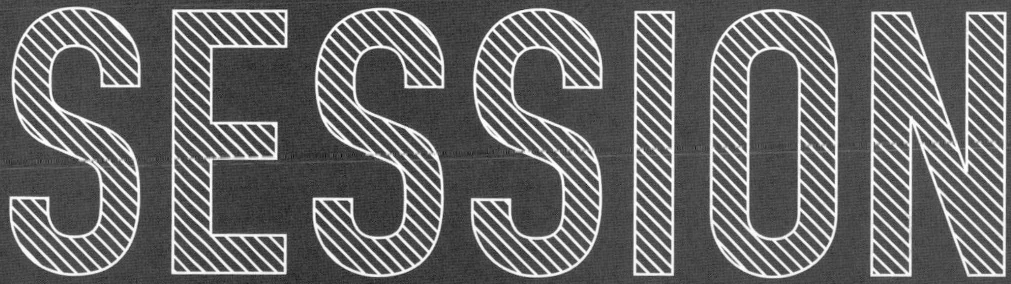

(Questions & Alli)

. Q&A .

QUESTIONS AND ALLI

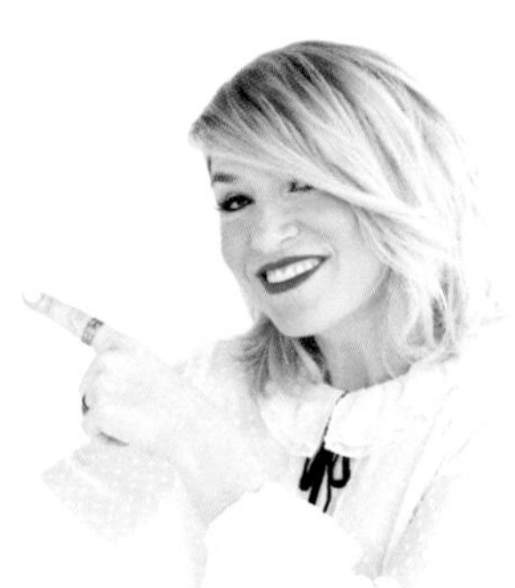

I gotta say, by this point in the book, I hope most of your burning questions about blow-drying your hair have been answered. However, that doesn't mean we're done here just yet.

1. **Why does my hair get greasy so fast?**
   Could be a few things. It could be that you naturally produce a fair amount of oil and might benefit from a double wash once in a while. Or maybe you didn't rinse your conditioner completely out. But one common cause of hair feeling greasy before its time is overdoing it with product. With the exception of volumizing products, most styling aids should not be used near your root area. When they are, natural oils from your scalp plus whatever you are using add up to that greasy feeling you're talking about.

   P.S. Overwashing will also make your hair produce more oil. Try to wash at least every other day.

2. **How do I get volume in my hair?**
   It's all in the technique. There are many ways to achieve volume, but most important, you have to blow it in from wet to dry to set the hair. See Southern Comfort, page 109, for more details (this is a big one!).

3. **What can I do if my hair gets rained on?**
   For rainy days, toss your favorite pomade or hair cream in your bag. If your hair gets wet or the humidity kicks in, take a small amount of product, rub it between your fingers, and start twisting 1- to 2-inch (2.5- to 5-cm) sections around your head. It's like a Mai Tai!

4. **My hair is so staticky. What do I do?**
   At home, sleeping on a silk pillowcase will help a lot. When you're out and about, tone down static with a couple swipes of a fabric softener sheet. Seriously, it works. If you have hair spray handy, spray a bit on your fingertips and smooth down those antennae.

5. **How do I combat frizz?**
   Well, first and foremost, make sure your hair is 100 percent dry, smooth, and sealed before you walk out the door. If your hair is even a little damp, it is sure to frizz up over the course of the day. Also, try to keep a travel-size hair spray, pomade, or cream in your purse—product is your hero when it comes to fighting frizz.

6. **My hair constantly feels dry. Is there anything that will help?**
   Treatments, treatments, treatments! Treatments are the answer. And there are so many options for you to choose from! Try an overnight hydrating mask two or three times a week: Apply the mask to damp hair, comb or brush product through, then pop on a shower cap. I use our Morning After Shower Cap—and turn it inside out so that the plastic is on the inside and the terry cloth is on the outside.

   Go as long between washes as you can so your scalp's natural oils can work their magic. When you do wash, condition with reparative hydrator like the Bay Breeze Hydrating Shot every time.

   Finally, use hydrating products before you blow-dry. Lightweight leave-in conditioners and heat protectants help your hair stand up to hot tools.

7. **How the heck am I supposed to style my bangs?**
   The trick to bangs is to first blow them dry holding your brush vertically, then sweep them back and forth across your forehead to create natural movement.

8. **How can I stop the flyaways around my face and part when hair spray doesn't totally solve that problem?**
   Flyaways, or, as I like to call them, antennae, come from overworking your bangs or overstretching very wet hair. We all have baby hairs, especially around the face, so always rough-dry the roots a little to allow those baby hairs to settle down, then grab your brush to start styling.

9. **My round brush always gets stuck in my hair. What gives?**
   Are your sections small enough? I can't stress enough the importance of working in clean 1- to 2-inch (2.5- to 5-cm) sections and making sure the hair on the brush isn't exceeding the size of the brush barrel. Perfecting each section before moving on to the next is the absolute key to a great, no-frizz blowout.

10. **How frequently should you trim your hair if you want to grow it out?**
    This is an age-old debate. I say trim it—and by trim I mean a very slight dusting—every four to six weeks. You don't want those frayed ends snapping off every time you blow out your hair.

11. **What should I do to protect my hair when I work out? I can't stand when it gets that dry, coarse feeling!**
    Detox Dry conditioner—because it has oils in it, it will keep your hair feeling soft and fresh.

12. **How important is it to have clean hair before a blowout?**
    It is everything. Everything. If your hair has lingering dirt or residue, then it won't blow out well and you'll have zero chance of hair with bounce and body. So. Sad.

13. **How hot is too hot for the flat iron?**
    I think a good rule of thumb with all tools is to keep the heat on a lower setting (300 to 350°F / 150 to 175°C) if your hair is damaged or very processed. Make sure you always use a heat protectant and don't leave an iron in your hair for more than a few seconds.

14. **How can I make my hair look better when I'm on vacation? I like to travel light!**
    This is when you must have the ideal products for your hair type. A sea-salt spritzer is great for straight hair that needs some hold and texture, while shine cream, pomade, or hair oil helps calm and control unruly hair. One trick I love is twisting product into 1- to 2-inch (2.5- to 5-cm) sections of damp hair all around my head and then letting it dry completely. Once it has set, I use my fingers to gently tousle my hair and loosen up the look.

    And always pack a few bobby pins, so you can do a side braid or twist when hair feels out of control.

15. **How do I deal with a bad haircut?**
    You go to Drybar. Religiously. A great blowout can always camouflage a bad haircut. I've been doing hair for twenty-plus years and I have seen a lot of bad haircuts, but I'm telling you, having a professional stylist blow out your hair will not only help it look its best, but the stylist will see you and your hair differently than you do. They may change the part or switch it up in a way you haven't tried or even dreamed of. It's worth a shot, right?

16. **How do you fix a weird kink or texture issue post-styling? There's always that one piece of hair that won't cooperate!**
    Oh man, we have all been there. It's pretty darn hard to change dry hair without a hot tool, but you can try a few tricks:

    1. Wet only that area with water or a primer spray (which is much better for your hair) and re-blow it.

2. Try using a pomade, styling cream, or hair oil on your hands, and twist the funky sections until they've been camouflaged.
3. Always keep a few bobby pins around in case you can hide a frizzy spot by twisting in a braid or twist.

17. What's the difference between a curl and a wave?
I think of a curl as a spiral, like fusilli pasta. It can be a tight ringlet or loose and bouncy. I think of a wave as a loose S, more like a wide egg noodle. (Now, I'm hungry!)

18. How can I let my hair air-dry naturally and still have it look good?
For us curly/wavy/frizzy ladies, there are definitely ways to make your hair look great without blowing it out. It's all about using the right product and setting your hair while it's wet. It might take you a few times to find your product combo, but for me, I gravitate toward products that will help calm and soften my hair—like a super lightweight leave-in conditioner (focusing application on my ends) or a hair primer. After I apply product and comb it through, I tousle it and let it air-dry for few minutes. Then I usually mist it all over with sea salt spray like Mai Tai Spritzer for texture and start twisting 1-inch (2.5-cm) sections all over. You want to make sure you get all your hair loosely twisted. Once in a while, I'll twist in a little hydrating control cream like Chaser to help tame the frizz. Now comes the most important part:

DO NOT TOUCH THE TWISTED SECTIONS UNTIL YOUR HAIR IS COMPLETELY DRY!

Once your hair is completely dry, softly and gently break up some of the twisted sections and tousle with your fingers. If there is still some lingering frizz, use cream or pomade and re-twist those sections. You'll end up with your very own variation of a Mai Tai.

19. **How do you get those fantabulous bangs of yours to stay in place?**
    Aw shucks! Thanks. I like to call it my swoop and I am proud of it! It's all about the blowout and the way you hold your brush: It must be vertical, never horizontal. We talk about this on page 80.

    And you know you can ask me anything, right? Find me on Instagram and Twitter at @alliwebb and @thedrybar. I'll always do my very best to get back to you.

20. **What do I do if I'm too tired for any of this stuff?**
    Head to your nearest Drybar ;)

10 CORE VALUES

RAISING THE DRYBAR

Drybar is bigger than just blowouts. When Cam, Michael, Sarah, and I started this company, I knew it was about more than having a good hair day, but I had no idea of the incredible impact and confidence boost gorgeous hair could provide. I'm so proud that our sole focus and purpose are to help women look and, more important, feel their absolute best.

We are big ole believers in promoting positivity and happiness, and just love it when we can brighten someone's day—for no particular reason. As we grew, we wanted to find a way to hold on to these ideals no matter what, and share them with all the amazing people who have come along on this ride. So we came up with our ten core values and beliefs. I'm so honored and humbled to share them with you!

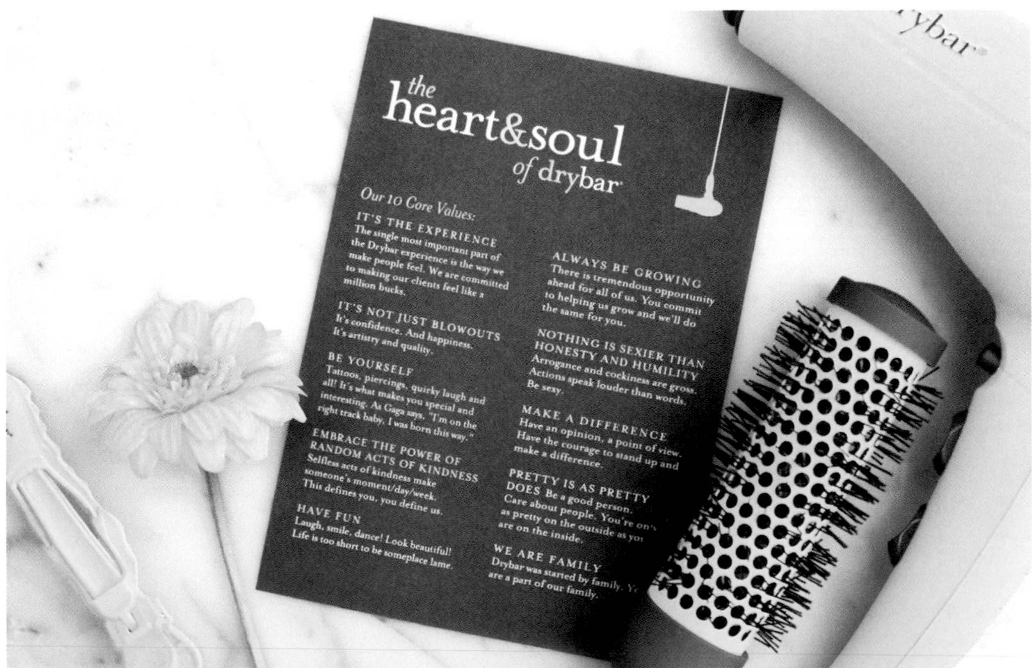

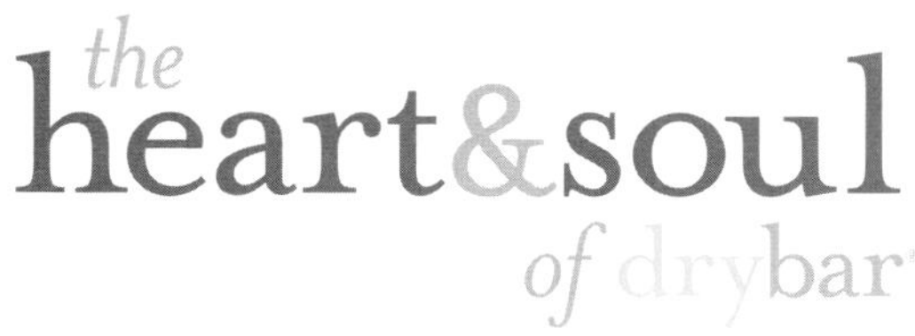

1. **It's the Experience**
   The single most important part of the Drybar experience is the way we make people feel. We are committed to making our clients—and anyone reading this book!—feel like a million bucks.

2. **It's Not Just the Blowout**
   It's the confidence and happiness that come from a great blowout.

3. **Be Yourself**
   Tattoos, piercings, quirky laugh, and all! It's what makes you special and interesting. Let people see the real you.

4. **Embrace the Power of Random Acts of Kindness**
   Selfless acts of kindness make someone's moment/day/week. It's these magical, unexpected moments that can change the course of everything.

5. **Have Fun**
   Laugh, smile, dance! Look beautiful! Life is too short to waste time being bored or lame.

6. **Always Be Growing**
   There is tremendous opportunity ahead for all of us. Whether or not you are at Drybar, you have the chance to make the most of each and every day.

7. **Nothing is Sexier Than Honesty and Humility**
   Actions speak louder than words. Be sexy.

8. **Make a Difference**
   Have an opinion, a point of view. Have the courage to stand up and make a difference.

9. **Pretty Is As Pretty Does**
   As my dad always said, you're only as pretty on the outside as you are on the inside. You might have amazing hair, but no one is going to want to sit with you if you've got a crummy attitude, so be nice. It looks good on you.

10. **We Are Family**
    Drybar was started by family. You are a part of our family. We wouldn't be where we are without you.

THANK YOU

TO CAM:

To my biggest cheerleader, my greatest advisor, my best friend and my heart, Cameron Webb. For without him, Drybar would not be Drybar.

Thank you, Cam, for being my amazingly patient husband and the creative mastermind and gatekeeper of the Drybar brand. I have learned so much from you over the years, but mostly, I have learned to just sit back and watch his genius. Your mind works in magical ways I'll never understand. I admire your dedication and work ethic (but hate that you get home so late all the time!). You are also arguably the world's best father to Grant and Kit, our super energetic and wonderful boys. I'm eternally grateful for your love, crazy humor, and kindness. Cam, I'll love you forever.

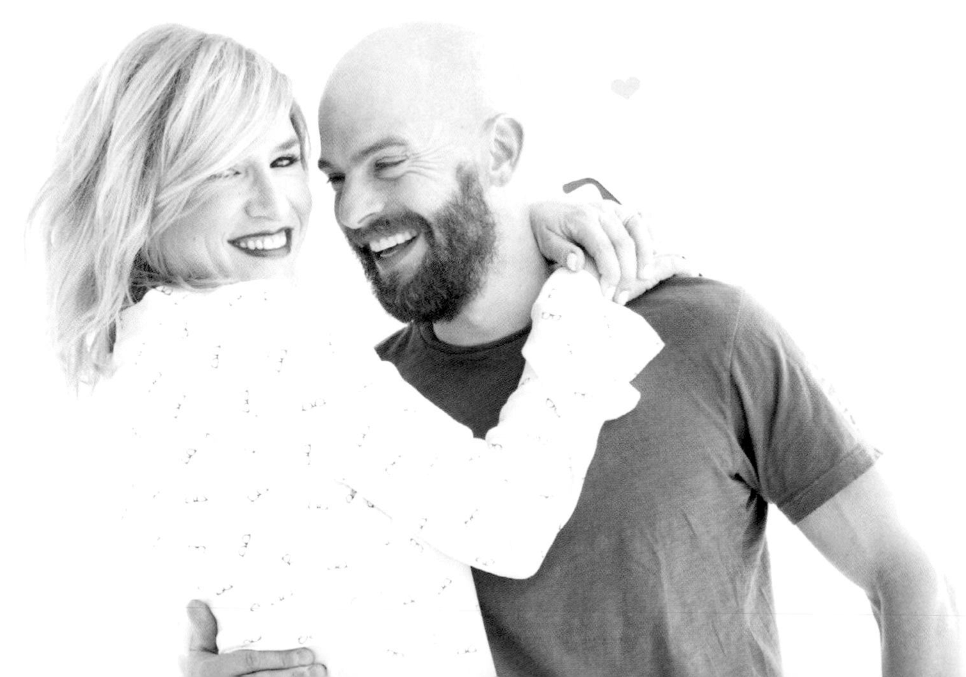

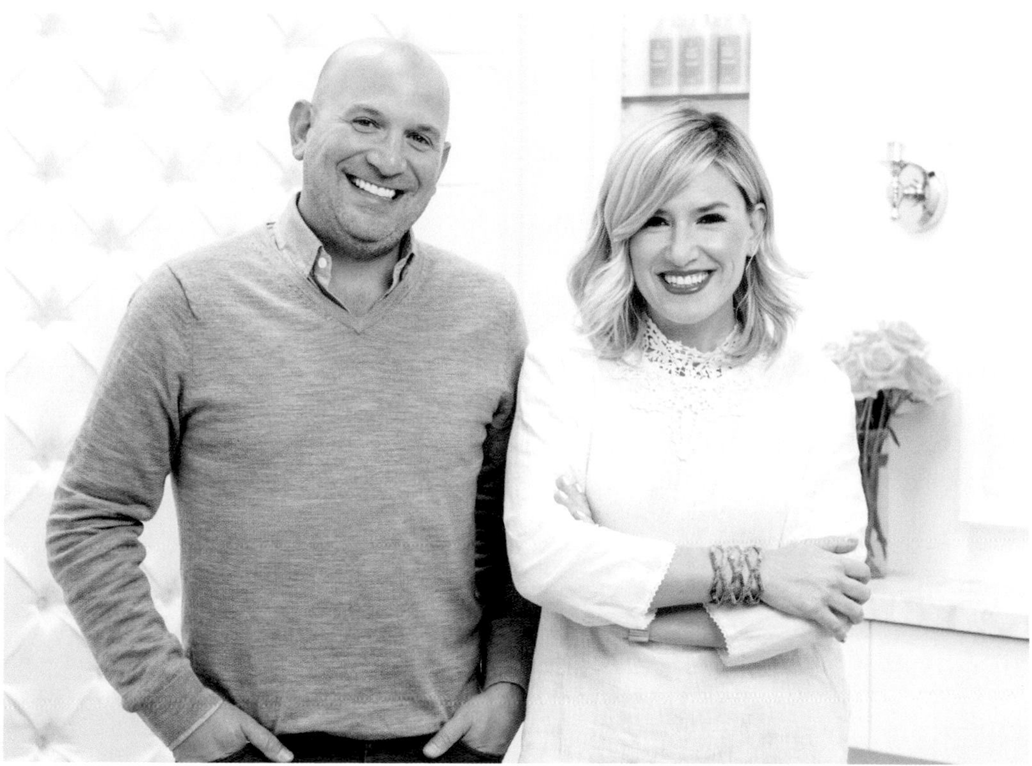

TO MICHAEL:

We have been thick as thieves my entire life and I owe so much of who I am today to you, Michael Landau. You have played so many crucial roles for me including being the overprotective big brother, an incredible mentor, and more recently the guy who keeps me in check. I love you to the moon and back.

Our friendship and bond is truly unbreakable. I don't think we ever thought we'd find such success together, but boy, am I grateful to be working together on this dream-come-true, once-in-a-lifetime opportunity. Besides being my own personal Google, you are my best friend and my mentor. Thank you for putting up with me all these years. I love you more than all the stars in the sky.

TO MY DAD:

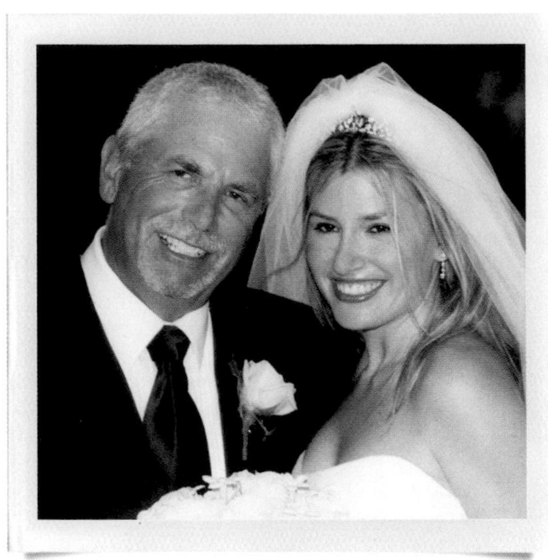

I couldn't publish this book without thanking my adoring father, Phil Landau.

Dad, your voice is always in my head and I am so grateful for all the wonderful life lessons you taught me as I was growing up (and for always noticing my hair!). You made me understand that beauty on the inside is way more important than beauty on the outside.

Thank you for always believing in me and knowing I would make the right decisions . . . and for giving me your naturally curly hair, for without that, Drybar would never have been born.

I love you more than words can ever say.

TO SARAH LANDAU:

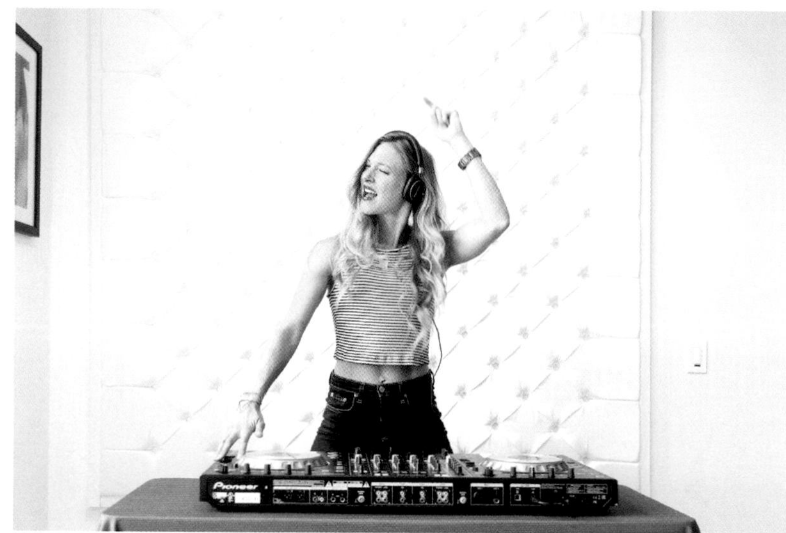

To Sarah, the sister I never had. The last six years have been quite the adventure for us. I'll never forget those first few months in Brentwood when we spent every second in the shop day after day, night after night. Living the Drybar dream! It was such a special time that I couldn't have survived without you. I know I speak for the entire Drybar family when I say thank you for bringing happiness to everyone around you through your music and spirit! I'll always be envious of your naturally straight hair, but still love you tons!

A SPECIAL MESSAGE TO ALL OUR INCREDIBLE DRYBAR STYLISTS:

I want to take a moment to send out a big hug and an even bigger thank-you to each and every one of you. Plain and simple, Drybar would not be what it has become without you guys. I am continually humbled, impressed, and inspired by your talent, creativity, and commitment to our cause.

Almost seven years ago, I started interviewing stylists (by having them blow out my crazy hair again and again!) in the living room of my little house in West Los Angeles. I remember being so worried that I wouldn't be able to find enough stylists who, like me, truly loved the styling part of hair. I posted an ad on Craigslist and wondered if anyone would call. Well, you did, and you keep showing up and joining our very special family.

You have made my dreams come true. From the bottom of my heart, thank you.

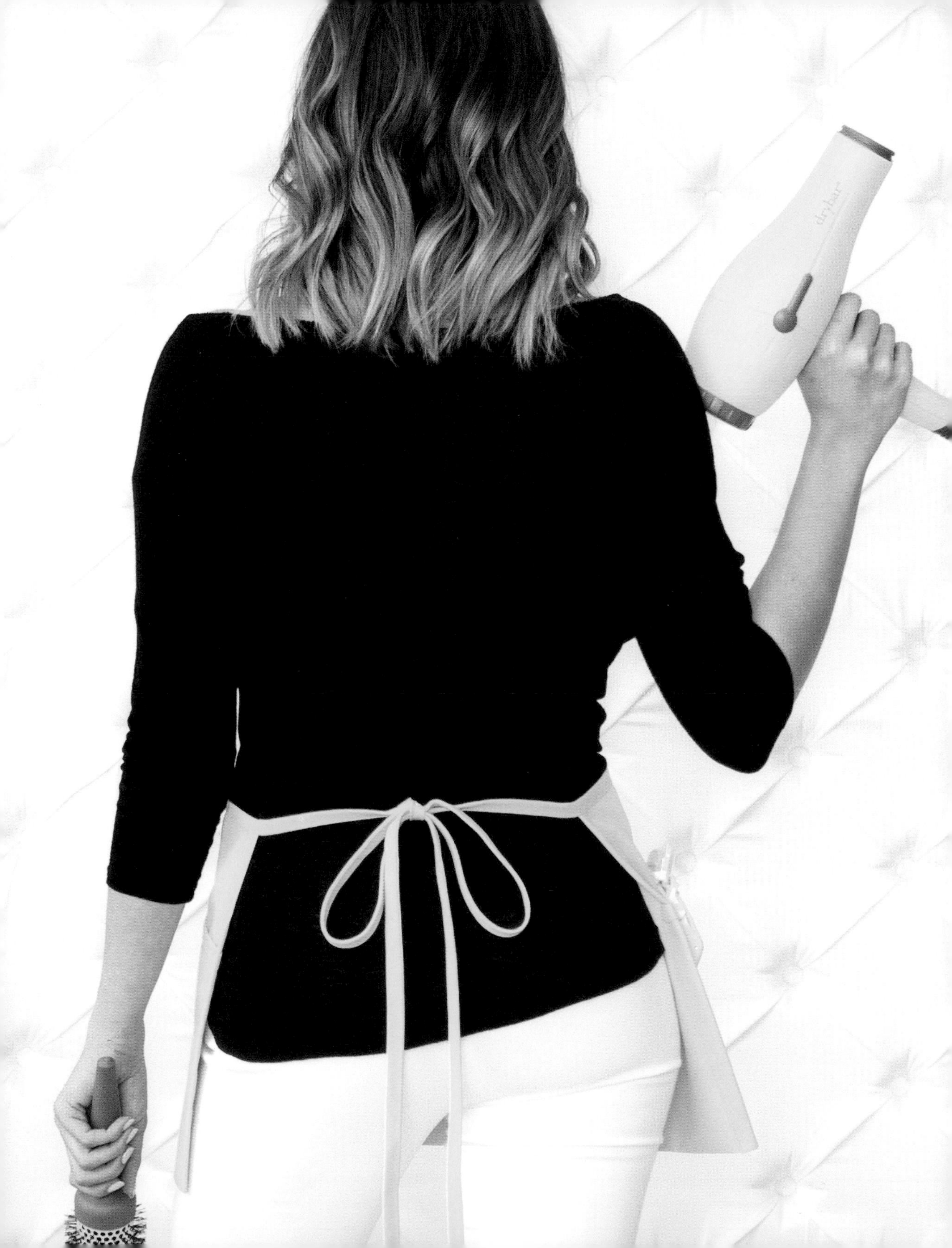
drybar

ACKNOWLEDGMENTS

THERE ARE COUNTLESS PEOPLE WHO HAVE HELPED MAKE DRYBAR WHAT IT IS TODAY.

For starters, our incredible architect and designer, Josh Heitler, who came up with the original Drybar prototype, and has helped craft every single shop since. And the team at Castanea Partners, led by Steve Berg, Janet Gurwitch, and Adam Garcia Eveloff, who stepped in to not only pay for all those beautiful shops but have also shared a tremendous amount of guidance and wisdom that has been invaluable in helping build this business. We could not have asked for better partners.

And then there are the true stars: My incredible and talented 3,000+ stylists, our stellar shop managers and educators, and our team of 70+ truly dedicated professionals who work tirelessly behind the scenes at our Support Center. They are all led by our fearless leader, John Heffner. Coming into a "family business" could be a challenge for most, but John, we cannot thank you enough for how thoughtfully and respectfully you've worked with us to build the foundation for Drybar's bright future.

So it turns out, writing a book is really hard! I'm incredibly indebted to a whole bunch of fantastic people who helped sculpt this book into something beautiful and amazing. I'm so grateful for these very special people in my corner:

Crystal Meers
I mean, it really doesn't get much better than you. You are an eternal ray of sunshine and happiness wrapped up in extraordinary talent. I feel so lucky to know you and to have had the honor of working with you on this crazy hair journey of ours. I'm pretty sure you now know how to perfect any blowout. Thank you a million times over for your patience, wisdom, insights, and warmth.

Tessa "Marchetti" Johnson
Thank you for your unending passion and excitement around this project. Not only did you make sure every little detail was taken care of, you made the entire process seamless and fun. You are a very special lady and I love working so closely with you.

Andrea Rell
You are my forever cheerleader and creative guru. Laughing, singing, and being ridiculously silly together is a something I will always cherish. Thank you for always being straight with me, the late nights at my house, and for sharing my office.

Julie Parks
My most trusted hair confidant. Watching you grow over the last five years has been an absolute joy. I'm so grateful for all your help on this book and for always being my extra set of eyes.

Katherine LaCroix
You run my life and do it with a smile. I'm so thankful to you for putting up with me and my crazy schedule 24/7.

Ashley Duckworth
Where would we be without you? I truly love working so closely with you as our director of training and I can't ever thank you enough for always indulging my requests, no matter how crazy or last minute they are! And, by the way, we actually can have nice things.

BrandLink Communications
Can't thank you all enough for the endless hard work, late nights, and extreme dedication, not only to this book, but for all you do for us every day.

Max Wanger
Your talent is endless. Thank you so much for making this book look so beautiful and for the creating the best shoots ever, even when it involves a skateboarding accident. Here's to many more great pics together.

Olive & June
Our nails never looked better! Huge thanks to my girl Sarah Gibson Tuttle for always being so generous and a seriously kick-ass mom, business owner, and incredible friend.

Too Faced Make-Up
Big thanks for the gorgeous makeup! We all fell in love with the incredible Tommie Rocha—she made us look flawless and glowy day after day.

Kristyn Keene & Kari Stuart at ICM
Forever grateful to you for holding my hand and explaining every step of the way with so much patience and ease.

Rebecca Kaplan and the Abrams Team
Thank you for believing in me and this little hair book of mine. You made this a truly wonderful experience.

To Papa John
A big thanks to you for all your support and partnership (and for being the only adult in the room!). Drybar wouldn't be where it is without you and your leadership. We are all better for knowing you.